W9-AFG-567

Diabetes Slow Cooker Recipes

Judith Finlayson

Barbara Selley, BA, RD
Nutrition Editor

Robert
ROSE

Diabetes Slow Cooker Recipes
Text copyright © 2007 Judith Finlayson
Photographs copyright © 2007 Robert Rose Inc.
Cover and text design copyright © 2007 Robert Rose Inc.

No part of this publication may be reproduced, stored in a retrieval system or transmitted, in any form or
by any means, without the prior written consent of the publisher or a licence from the Canadian Copyright
Licensing Agency (Access Copyright). For an Access Copyright licence, visit www.accesscopyright.ca or
call toll-free: 1-800-893-5777.

For complete cataloguing information, see page 248.

Disclaimer

The recipes in this book have been carefully tested by our kitchen and our tasters. To the best of our knowledge,
they are safe and nutritious for ordinary use and users. For those people with food or other allergies, or who have
special food requirements or health issues, please read the suggested contents of each recipe carefully and
determine whether or not they may create a problem for you. All recipes are used at the risk of the consumer.

We cannot be responsible for any hazards, loss or damage that may occur as a result of any recipe use.

For those with special needs, allergies, requirements or health problems, in the event of any doubt, please
contact your medical adviser prior to the use of any recipe.

Design & Production: Joseph Gisini/PageWave Graphics Inc.

Editor: Sue Sumeraj

Index: Belle Wong

Photography: Colin Erricson

Food Stylists: Kate Bush and Kathy Robertson

Props Stylist: Charlene Erricson

Cover image: Moroccan-Style Lamb with Raisins and Apricots (see recipe, page 216)

We acknowledge the financial support of the Government of Canada through the Book Publishing Industry
Development Program (BPIDP) for our publishing activities.

Published by: Robert Rose Inc.
120 Eglinton Ave. E., Suite 800, Toronto, Ontario, Canada M4P 1E2
Tel: (416) 322-6552 Fax: (416) 322-6936

Printed in Canada

1 2 3 4 5 6 7 8 9   CPL   15 14 13 12 11 10 09 08 07

Contents

Acknowledgments

Once again, my thanks to the great creative team who works behind the scenes to ensure that my books achieve the highest degree of excellence in editing, photography, styling and design: all the folks at PageWave Graphics — Andrew Smith, Joseph Gisini, Kevin Cockburn and Daniella Zanchetta — for their great design work; my editor, Sue Sumeraj, who consistently notices things that I miss; Kate Bush and Charlene Erricson for their talented styling; and last, but certainly not least, Mark Shapiro and Colin Erricson for their beautiful photographs, which make my recipes look delicious.

Special thanks to Barbara Selley, RD, whose work on the diabetes-specific aspects of this book has been amazingly thorough and consistently professional. And thanks to the volunteer health professionals at the CDA who reviewed the book.

I'd also like to thank Audrey King and Jennifer MacKenzie for their diligent help with recipe testing and all my friends and neighbors who gallantly tuck in to my culinary creations, even those that miss the mark, and provide thoughtful comments that are always useful in fine-tuning the end result.

Thanks also to Bob Dees and Marian Jarkovich at Robert Rose for their consistent commitment to ensuring that my books are well received in the marketplace.

Introduction

This is my sixth slow cooker cookbook. The more I use my slow cooker, the more ideas I have for using this versatile appliance. It fits so well with how I like to cook that I'm constantly seeing new ways to incorporate its services into my life. So, perhaps not surprisingly, I became interested in finding ways to combine the burgeoning interest in health and nutrition with the convenience of using a slow cooker.

Like most people, I'm becoming increasingly aware of the important role diet plays in health. By habitually eating an assortment of foods from all the food groups, you're making sure you get the *range* of nutrients you need.

Planning what and when you will eat is especially important for people with diabetes. You need to

- take time for breakfast;

- eat each day a variety of foods from all the food groups — grains, preferably whole grains, vegetables, fruits, milk and alternatives, and meat and alternatives;

- choose appropriate portions;

- space meals 4 to 6 hours apart; and

- snack only if you and your dietitian and other health care providers decide it is necessary for good blood glucose control.

For people with diabetes, one of the primary goals is maintaining or achieving a healthy weight. This means controlling calorie intake and limiting total fat to no more than 30% of calories and saturated fat to no more than 10% of calories.[1] For a person eating 2,000 calories a day, for example, the total fat consumed should be about 65 grams, including no more than 22 grams of saturated fat.

Controlling sodium is also important. Sodium in the diet comes primarily from salt, whether it be used in cooking, added at the table or hidden in manufactured and prepared foods. Consider that one teaspoon (5 mL) of salt contains about 2,400 mg of sodium. The American Diabetes Association limits sodium to 2,400–6,000 mg per day, while the Canadian Diabetes Association suggests 2,000–4,000 mg. In both cases, the lower end of the range is recommended.[2]

There is a common misconception that those with diabetes should avoid carbohydrates, especially sugar. This is not true, but you should control the total amount of

[1] Canadian Diabetes Association, "2003 Clinical Practice Guidelines for the Prevention and Management of Diabetes in Canada," *Can J Diabetes* 27, Suppl. no. 2 (2003): S21–S23.

[2] American Diabetes Association, "Standards of Medical Care in Diabetes — 2006," *Diabetes Care* 29 (2006): S4–S42; Canadian Diabetes Association, "2003 Clinical Practice Guidelines for the Prevention and Management of Diabetes in Canada," *Can J Diabetes* 27, Suppl. no. 2 (2003): S21–S23.

carbohydrate eaten and spread it evenly throughout the day's meals and snacks. Glycemic index, a scale that ranks carbohydrate-rich foods by how fast and how much they raise blood glucose, is also important. Foods such as legumes, vegetables and whole-grain foods have a lower glycemic index and should be consumed often. To learn more about glycemic index, consult your diabetes educator or visit **www.diabetes.ca** or **www.diabetes.org**.

A slow cooker makes it much easier to plan and prepare in advance and to have meals on the table on time. I've included a wide range of recipes, from hearty soups to elegant desserts, most accompanied by Make Ahead information to help you take full advantage of the convenience provided by a slow cooker.

The recipes

- emphasize healthy servings of whole grains, legumes, vegetables and fruit;

- generally provide, per serving, not more than 35 grams of carbohydrate, 3 Meat Exchanges/3 Meat and Alternatives Choices, and 10 grams of fat;

- contain moderate amounts of salt (less than 800 mg of sodium per serving, and often much less); and

- call for non-hydrogenated fats and oils.

Commercially produced trans fats, which have a well-documented adverse effect on cardiovascular health, should be avoided and, whenever possible, saturated fats should be replaced with unsaturated fats, which have numerous health benefits. To help you get the most out of this book, in addition to the total amount of fat per serving, saturated, monounsaturated and polyunsaturated fat are also reported.

Vegetarian and vegan recipes are labeled as such.

I hope you will find this book helpful. More importantly, I hope you will use it often to get the most out of the convenience your slow cooker provides by preparing delicious and nutritious meals that help to keep you and yours happy and well.

— Judith Finlayson

Using Your Slow Cooker

The slow cooker's less-is-better approach is, in many ways, the secret of its success. The appliance does its work by cooking foods very slowly — from about 200°F (90°C) on the Low setting to 300°F (150°C) on High. This slow, moist cooking environment enables the appliance to produce mouthwatering braises, chilies and many other kinds of soups and stews, as well as delicious breakfast cereals and desserts.

An Effective Time Manager

In addition to producing great-tasting food, a slow cooker is one of the most effective time-management tools available. Most recipes can be at least partially prepared up to two days before you intend to cook. (For detailed instructions, look for the Make Ahead that accompanies appropriate recipes.) Once the ingredients have been assembled in the stoneware and the appliance is turned on, you can pretty much forget about it. The slow cooker performs unattended while you carry on with your workaday life. You can be away from the kitchen all day and return to a hot, delicious meal.

A Low-Tech Appliance

Slow cookers are amazingly low tech. The appliance usually consists of a metal casing and a stoneware insert with a tight-fitting lid. For convenience, this insert should be removable from the metal casing, making it easier to clean and increasing its versatility as a serving dish. The casing contains the heat source: electric coils that usually surround the stoneware insert. These coils do their work using the energy it takes to power a 100-watt light bulb. Because the slow cooker operates on such a small amount of energy, you can safely leave it turned on while you are away from home.

Slow Cooker Basics

Slow cookers are generally round or oval and range in size from 1 to 7 quarts. I feel there is a benefit to having two: a smaller (3- to 4-quart) one, which is ideal for making recipes with smaller yields, such as breakfast cereals and some desserts; and a larger (6-quart) oval one, which is necessary for cooking larger quantities, as well as for making recipes that call for setting a baking dish or pan inside the stoneware. Because the heating coils usually surround the stoneware, most slow cookers cook from the sides, rather than the bottom, which means you'll produce better results if the stoneware is at least half-full. Some manufacturers sell a "slow cooker" that is actually a multi-cooker. It has a heating element at the bottom and, in my experience, it cooks faster than a traditional slow cooker. Also, since the heat source is at the bottom, it is likely that the food will scorch during the long cooking time unless it is stirred.

Your slow cooker should come with a booklet that explains how to use the appliance. I recommend that you read this carefully and/or visit the manufacturer's website for specific information on the model you purchased. I've cooked with a variety of slow cookers and have found that cooking times can vary substantially from one to another. Although it may not seem particularly helpful if you're just starting out, the only firm advice I can give is: Know your slow cooker. After trying a few of these recipes, you will get a sense of whether your slow cooker is faster or slower than the ones I use, and you will be able to adjust the cooking times accordingly.

Other variables that can affect cooking time are extreme humidity, power fluctuations and high altitudes. Be extra vigilant if any of these circumstances affect you.

Slow Cooker Tips

Like all appliances, the slow cooker has its unique way of doing things and, as a result, you need to understand how it works and adapt your cooking style accordingly. Success in the slow cooker, like success in the oven or on top of the stove, depends on using proper cooking techniques. The slow cooker saves you time because it allows you to forget about the food once it is in the stoneware. But you must still pay attention to the advance preparation. Here are a few tips that will help ensure slow cooker success.

Soften Vegetables

Although it requires using an extra pan, I am committed to softening most vegetables before adding them to the slow cooker. In my experience, this is not the most time-consuming part of preparing a slow cooker dish — it usually takes longer to peel and chop the vegetables, which you have to do anyway. But softening vegetables such as onions and carrots dramatically improves the quality of the dish for two reasons: it adds color and begins the process of caramelization, which breaks down the vegetables' natural sugars and releases their flavor; and it extracts the fat-soluble components of foods, which further enriches the taste. Moreover, tossing herbs and spices with the softened vegetables emulsifies their flavor, helping to produce a sauce in which the flavors are better integrated into the dish than they would have been if this step had been skipped.

Reduce Liquid

As you use your slow cooker, one of the first things you will notice is that it generates a tremendous amount of liquid. Because slow cookers cook at a low heat, tightly covered, liquid doesn't evaporate as it does in the oven or on top of the stove. As a result, food made from traditional recipes will be watery. So the second rule of successful slow cooking is to reduce the amount of liquid. Naturally, you don't want to reduce the flavor, so I suggest using lower-salt broth or homemade salt-free stock, rather than water, to cook most of the dishes. The other potential problem with liquid generation is that it can affect the results of starch dishes, such as cakes and some grains. One technique that works well with such dishes is to place folded tea towels over top of the stoneware before covering with the lid. This prevents accumulated moisture from dripping onto the food.

Cut Root Vegetables into Thin Slices or Small Pieces

Perhaps surprisingly, root vegetables — carrots, parsnips, turnips and, particularly, potatoes — cook very slowly in the slow cooker. As a result, root vegetables should be thinly sliced or cut into small pieces no larger than 1-inch (2.5 cm) cubes.

Pay Attention to Cooking Temperature

Many desserts, such as those containing milk, cream or some leavening agents, need to be cooked on High. In these recipes, a Low setting is not suggested as an option. For recipes that aren't dependent upon cooking at a particular temperature, the rule of thumb is that 1 hour of cooking on High equals 2 to $2\frac{1}{2}$ hours on Low.

Don't Overcook

Although slow cooking reduces your chances of overcooking food, it is still not a "one size fits all" solution to meal preparation. Many vegetables, such as beans, lentils and root vegetables, need a good 8-hour cooking span and may even benefit from a longer cooking time. But others, such as green beans and cauliflower, are usually cooked within 6 hours on Low and will be overcooked and unappetizing if left for longer. One solution (which, because of food safety concerns, is not possible if you are cooking meat) is to extend the cooking time by assembling the dish ahead, then refrigerating it overnight in the stoneware. Because the mixture and the stoneware are chilled, the vegetables will take longer to cook. This is a useful technique if you are cooking more-tender vegetables and need to be away from the house all day.

Use Ingredients Appropriately

Some ingredients do not respond well to long, slow cooking at all, and should be added during the last 30 minutes of cooking, after the temperature has been increased to High. These include zucchini, peas, snow peas, fish and seafood, as well as milk and cream (which will curdle if cooked too long.)

Although I love to cook with peppers, I've learned that most peppers become bitter if cooked for too long. The same holds true for cayenne pepper, hot pepper sauces (such as Tabasco) and large quantities of spicy curry powder (small quantities of mild curry powder seem to fare well, possibly because natural sugars in the vegetables counter any bitterness). The solution to this problem is to add fresh green or red bell peppers to recipes during the last 30 minutes of cooking, use cayenne pepper in small quantities, if at all, and add hot pepper sauce after the dish is cooked. All of the recipes in this book address these concerns in the instructions.

Tip

Many of the recipes call for 1/2 to 1 tsp (5 to 10 mL) of salt. In most cases, this could be omitted to reduce sodium intake.

Use Whole-Leaf Herbs and Coarsely Ground Spices

Spices (such as cumin seeds) that have been toasted and coarsely ground and whole-leaf herbs (such as dried thyme and oregano leaves) release their flavors slowly throughout the long cooking period. Finely ground spices and herbs, on the other hand, tend to lose flavor during slow cooking. If you're using fresh herbs, finely chop them — unless you're using the whole stem (which works best with thyme and rosemary) — and add during the last hour of cooking.

I recommend the use of cracked black peppercorns rather than ground pepper in many of my recipes because they release flavor slowly during the long cooking process. "Cracked pepper" can be purchased in the spice section of supermarkets, but I like to make my own using a mortar and pestle. If you prefer to use ground black pepper, use one-quarter to half the amount of cracked black peppercorns called for in the recipe.

Find Dishes and Pans That Fit into Your Stoneware

Some recipes, notably breads, need to be cooked in an extra dish placed in the slow cooker stoneware. Not only will you need a large oval slow cooker for this purpose, but finding a dish or pan that fits into the stoneware can be a challenge. I've found several kinds of dishes that suit this purpose well: standard 7-inch (17.5 cm) square baking pans; 4-cup (1 L) and 6-cup (1.5 L) ovenproof baking dishes; 6-cup (1.5 L) soufflé dishes; and 8- by 4-inch (20 by 10 cm) loaf pans.

Before you decide to make a recipe that requires a baking dish, make sure you have a container that will fit into your stoneware. I've noted the size and dimensions of the containers used in all relevant recipes. Be aware that varying the size and shape of the dish is likely to affect cooking times.

Maximize Slow Cooker Convenience

In addition to producing mouthwatering food, a slow cooker's great strength is convenience. Where appropriate, my recipes contain a Make Ahead tip that will help you maximize this attribute. To get the most out of your slow cooker,

- Prepare ingredients to the cooking stage the night before you intend to cook, to keep work to a minimum in the morning.

- Cook a recipe overnight and refrigerate until ready to serve.

Serving Size Matters

In the 1970s, a typical pasta serving in a restaurant was 1 cup (250 mL); now, it's not unusual to see a serving size of 3 cups (750 mL). Bagels weighing 5 oz (150 g) or more dwarf those of 30 years ago, which were 2 to 3 oz (60 to 85 g).

We encounter this "portion distortion" or "portion creep" everywhere we turn. And it's easy to start choosing larger amounts of food than we need, often without realizing it. So you may find that some of the serving sizes in this book are smaller than you're accustomed to. The Portion Calculator on pages 13–15 will help you serve yourself the right amount.

Portion Calculator

Delicious aromas are wafting from your slow cooker, and dinner is ready. You know the recipe makes 8 servings, but how much is one serving?

Dishing up the right size serving from a large quantity in a slow cooker can be a challenge. But with a little one-time-only "homework," you'll always be able to determine how much food is in your slow cooker — and then your serving size. You'll need a measuring cup or a metric measure for liquids, and a ruler, preferably plastic or metal.

Using Imperial Measures

1. Count the number of measuring cups of water needed to fill the slow cooker stoneware one-half to three-quarters full.
2. Measure the depth of the water to the nearest quarter-inch.
3. Divide the number of cups by the depth of the water in inches to calculate the number of cups per inch.

Example

You've poured 12 cups of water into the stoneware of a 6-quart slow cooker, and measured the depth of the water as $2\frac{3}{4}$ inches (or 2.75 inches).

12 (cups) ÷ 2.75 (inches) = 4.4 (cups per inch)

4. Use the value you obtained in Step 3 to calculate a table of volumes for various depths (rounding to the nearest cup), as follows:

Example

Depth	x 4.4 = Volume
2.25 inches	10 cups
2.5 inches	11 cups
2.75 inches	12 cups
3 inches	13 cups
3.25 inches	14 cups

Keep this table handy for quick reference when you are preparing meals in your slow cooker.

5. After you have prepared a meal in your slow cooker, measure the depth of the food, then refer to your table of volumes to determine how many cups of food you have. Divide this number by the number of servings stated in the recipe to determine the size of a serving.

Example

You've prepared chili, and the recipe states that it makes 10 servings. You measure the depth of the chili and find that it is 3 inches deep. Referring to your handy table of volumes, you see that you have 13 cups of chili. You divide the number of cups (13) by the number of servings (10), and learn that each serving will be 1.3 cups (roughly $1\frac{1}{3}$ cups). This $1\frac{1}{3}$-cup serving will provide the nutrients and America's Exchanges/Canada's Choices stated in the recipe.

Using Metric Measures

1. Count the number of 250-mL measures of water needed to fill the slow cooker stoneware one-half to three-quarters full, then calculate the volume (in mL) of water currently held by the slow cooker:

Example
You've poured thirteen 250-mL measures of water into the stoneware of an 8-quart slow cooker.
13 x 250 = 3,250 mL

2. Measure the depth of the water to the nearest 0.5 cm.
3. Divide the volume of the water by the depth of the water in centimeters to calculate the number of mL per cm.

Example
You've calculated the volume of the water as 3,250 mL, and measured the depth of the water as 8 cm.
3,250 (mL) ÷ 8 (cm) = 406 mL per cm

4. Use the value you obtained in Step 3 to calculate a table of volumes for various depths, as follows:

Example

Depth	x 406 = Volume
6.5 cm	2,639 mL
7 cm	2,842 mL
7.5 cm	3,045 mL
8 cm	3,248 mL
8.5 cm	3,451 mL

Keep this table handy for quick reference when you are preparing meals in your slow cooker.

5. After you have prepared a meal in your slow cooker, measure the depth of the food, then refer to your table of volumes to determine how many mL of food you have. Divide this number by the number of servings stated in the recipe to determine the size of a serving.

Example
You've prepared soup, and the recipe states that it serves 12. You measure the depth of the soup and find that it is 7.5 cm deep. Referring to your handy table of volumes, you know that you therefore have 3,045 mL of soup. You divide this number by the serving size (12), and learn that each serving will be about 250 mL. This 250-mL serving will provide the nutrients and America's Exchanges/Canada's Choices stated in the recipe.

Tip

If you are refrigerating a slow cooker soup, chili or similar mixed dish for a later meal, measure out single-serving amounts into individual storage containers.

Food Safety in the Slow Cooker

Because it cooks at a very low temperature for long periods of time, cooking with a slow cooker requires a bit more vigilance about food safety than does cooking at higher temperatures. The slow cooker needs to strike a delicate balance between cooking slowly enough that it doesn't require your attention and fast enough to ensure that food reaches temperatures that are appropriate to inhibit bacterial growth. Bacteria grow rapidly at temperatures higher than 40°F (4°C) and lower than 140°F (60°C). Once the temperature reaches 165°F (74°C), bacteria are killed. Slow cooker manufacturers have designed the appliance to ensure that bacterial growth is not a concern. As long as the lid is left on and the food is cooked for the appropriate length of time, that temperature will be reached quickly enough to ensure food safety.

Unless you have made part of the recipe ahead and refrigerated it, most of the ingredients in my recipes are warm when added to the slow cooker (the meat has been browned and the sauce has been thickened on the stovetop), which adds a cushion of comfort to any potential concerns about food safety.

The following tips will help to ensure that utmost food safety standards are met:

- Keep food refrigerated until you are ready to cook. Bacteria multiply quickly at room temperature. Do not allow ingredients to rise to room temperature before cooking.

- Do not partially cook meat or poultry and refrigerate for subsequent cooking. If you're browning meat before adding it to the slow cooker, do so just before placing it in the slow cooker. When cooking meat, try to get it to a high temperature as quickly as possible.

- If cooking a large cut of meat, such as a pot roast, that has been added to the stoneware without being browned, set the temperature at High for at least 1 hour to accelerate the cooking process.

- If preparing ingredients in advance of cooking, refrigerate precooked meat, such as ground beef or sausage, in a separate container from vegetables. Assemble when ready to cook.

Tip

Leaving the lid on when you're slow cooking, particularly during the early stages, helps to ensure that bacteria-killing temperatures are reached in the appropriate amount of time.

- Pay attention to the Make Ahead instructions for those recipes that can be partially prepared in advance of cooking — they have been developed to address food safety issues.

- Do not put frozen meat, fish or poultry into a slow cooker. Unless otherwise instructed, thaw frozen food before adding it to the slow cooker. Frozen fruits and vegetables should usually be thawed under cold running water to separate before being added to recipes.

- Don't lift the lid while food is cooking. Each time the lid is removed, it takes about 20 minutes for the slow cooker to recover the lost heat. This increases the time it takes for the food to reach the "safe zone."

- If you are away and the power goes out, discard the food if it has not finished cooking. If the food has cooked completely, it should be safe for up to 2 hours.

- Refrigerate leftovers as quickly as possible.

- Do not reheat food in the slow cooker.

Testing for Safe Temperatures

If you are concerned that your slow cooker isn't cooking quickly enough to ensure food safety, try this simple test. Fill the stoneware insert with 8 cups (2 L) of cold water and set the temperature to Low for 8 hours. Using an accurate thermometer (and checking quickly, because the temperature drops when the lid is removed), ensure that the temperature of the water is 185°F (85°C). If the water has not reached that temperature, the slow cooker is not heating food fast enough to avoid food safety problems. If the temperature is significantly higher than that, the appliance is not cooking slowly enough to be used as a slow cooker.

Leftovers

Cooked food can be kept warm in the slow cooker for up to 2 hours. At that point, it should be transferred to small containers so that it cools as rapidly as possible, and then should be refrigerated or frozen. Because the appliance heats up so slowly, food should never be reheated in a slow cooker.

Nutrient Analysis

The nutrient analyses and accompanying America's Exchanges and Canada's Choices for the recipes were prepared by Food Intelligence (Toronto, Ontario) and Info Access (1988) Inc. (Don Mills, Ontario).

The calculations were based on

- Imperial measures and weights (except for food typically packaged and used in metric quantities).

- The smaller ingredient amount when there was a range.

- The first ingredient listed when there was a choice.

- The exclusion of optional ingredients and those in unspecified amounts or "to taste."

For additional information about diet and diabetes, visit

- www.diabetes.org

- www.diabetes.ca

Calculations of America's Exchanges were based on the American Diabetes Association food exchange values in the table below. In these calculations, fiber is included in the carbohydrate value.

NUTRIENTS PER EXCHANGE			
GROUPS/LISTS	CARBOHYDRATE (g)	PROTEIN (g)	FAT (g)
Carbohydrate Group			
Starch	15	3	0–1
Fruit	15	–	–
Milk			
Fat-free, low-fat	12	8	0–3
Reduced-fat	12	8	5
Whole	12	8	8
Other Carbohydrates	15	v*	v*
Vegetables	5	2	–
Meat and Meat Substitutes Group			
Very lean	–	7	0–1
Lean	–	7	3
Medium-fat	–	7	5
High-fat	–	7	8
Fat Group	–	–	5

* v = variable
Source: Adapted from *Exchange Lists for Meal Planning,* American Diabetes Association and American Dietetic Association, 2003.

Canada's Choices calculations were based on the Canadian Diabetes Association food choice values in the table below. Available carbohydrate (total amount less dietary fiber) is totaled for all ingredients and is reported as Carbohydrate Choices.

NUTRIENTS PER CHOICE			
CANADA'S CHOICES	CARBOHYDRATE (g)	PROTEIN (g)	FAT (g)
Carbohydrate	15	0	0
Grains & Starches	15	3	0
Fruits	15	1	0
Milk (1%) & Alternatives	15	8	2.5
Other Choices	15	v*	v*
Vegetables	<5 (most)	2	0
Meat and Alternatives	0	7	3–5
Fats	0	0	5
Extras	<5	0	0

* v = variable
Source: Adapted from *Beyond the Basics: Meal Planning, Healthy Eating and Diabetes Prevention and Management,* Version 2, Canadian Diabetes Association, December 20, 2005.

Breakfasts, Breads, Dips and Spreads

Hot Breakfast Cereals

MAKES 4 SERVINGS

Tip

Rolled oats, often called porridge when cooked, are probably the most popular breakfast cereal. For variety, try steel-cut oats, Irish oatmeal or Scotch oats, which have an appealing chewy texture.

Hot cereal is one of my favorite ways to begin the day, and happily, you can use your slow cooker to cook the cereal overnight. Just leave the slow cooker on Warm in the morning and everyone can help themselves.

- **These recipes work best in a small (maximum 3½ quart) slow cooker**
- **Greased slow cooker stoneware**

Hot Multigrain Cereal

1 cup	multigrain cereal, or ½ cup (125 mL) multigrain cereal and ½ cup (125 mL) rolled oats	250 mL
¼ tsp	salt	1 mL
4 cups	water	1 L
1	all-purpose apple, peeled and thickly sliced	1
	Wheat germ, optional	

1. In prepared slow cooker stoneware, combine multigrain cereal, salt, water and apple. Cover and cook on Low for 8 hours or overnight. Add wheat germ, if using. Stir well and serve.

Hot Oatmeal

1⅓ cups	rolled oats	325 mL
¼ tsp	salt	1 mL
4¼ cups	water	1.05 L
	Wheat germ, optional	

1. In prepared slow cooker stoneware, combine oats, salt and water. Cover and cook on Low for 8 hours or overnight. Add wheat germ, if using. Stir well and serve.

Mindful Morsels

Wheat germ is very nutrient-dense. Just 2 tsp (10 mL) is an excellent source of manganese and also supplies folacin, thiamine, magnesium and zinc.

Hot Multigrain Cereal

NUTRIENTS PER SERVING	
Calories	116
Fat	1.7 g
Saturates	0.0 g
Polyunsaturates	0.0 g
Monounsaturates	0.0 g
Cholesterol	0 mg
Sodium	148 mg
Carbohydrate	24.5 g
Fiber	5.5 g
Protein	3.9 g

Hot Oatmeal

NUTRIENTS PER SERVING	
Calories	120
Fat	2.1 g
Saturates	0.4 g
Polyunsaturates	0.8 g
Monounsaturates	0.7 g
Cholesterol	0 mg
Sodium	146 mg
Carbohydrate	21.1 g
Fiber	3.2 g
Protein	4.4 g

Hot Multigrain Cereal and Hot Oatmeal

AMERICA'S EXCHANGES		CANADA'S CHOICES	
1½	Starch	1	Carbohydrate

MAKES 8 SERVINGS

Tips

Like lentils, some millet may contain bits of dirt or discolored grains. If your millet looks grimy, rinse it thoroughly in a pot of water before using. Swish it around and remove any offending particles, then rinse under cold running water.

This cereal tends to get dry and brown around the edges if cooked for longer than 8 hours. If you need to cook it for longer, add an additional 1/2 cup (125 mL) of water.

If you're not using Medjool dates, which are naturally soft, place the chopped dates in a microwave-safe dish, cover with water and microwave on High for 30 seconds to soften before adding to cereal.

Multigrain Cereal with Fruit

A steaming bowl of this tasty cereal will get you off to a good start in the morning.

- **Works best in a small (3 1/2 quart) slow cooker (see Tip, page 22)**
- **Greased slow cooker stoneware**

1/2 cup	brown rice	125 mL
1/2 cup	millet (see Tips, left)	125 mL
1/2 cup	wheat berries	125 mL
2	medium all-purpose apples, peeled, cored and thinly sliced	2
4 cups	water (see Tips, left)	1 L
1/2 tsp	vanilla	2 mL
1/2 cup	chopped pitted soft dates, preferably Medjool (see Tips, left)	125 mL
	Wheat germ, optional	

1. In prepared slow cooker stoneware, combine rice, millet, wheat berries and apples. Add water and vanilla. Cover and cook on Low for up to 8 hours or overnight. Add dates and stir well. Serve sprinkled with wheat germ, if using.

NUTRIENTS PER SERVING	
Calories	232
Fat	1.4 g
Saturates	0.2 g
Polyunsaturates	0.6 g
Monounsaturates	0.3 g
Cholesterol	0 mg
Sodium	9 mg
Carbohydrate	52.2 g
Fiber	6.1 g
Protein	5.0 g

AMERICA'S EXCHANGES	
2	Starch
1 1/2	Fruit

CANADA'S CHOICES	
3	Carbohydrate

MAKES 8 SERVINGS

Tip

If you are cooking this cereal in a large oval slow cooker, reduce the cooking time by half.

Apple Oatmeal with Wheat Berries

This flavorful cereal is an adaptation of a recipe that appeared in Eat, Drink and Be Healthy: The Harvard Medical School Guide to Healthy Eating.

- **Works best in a small (3½ quart) slow cooker (see Tip, left)**
- **Greased slow cooker stoneware**

1½ cups	steel-cut oats	375 mL
½ cup	wheat berries	125 mL
2	apples, peeled, cored and chopped	2
½ tsp	ground cinnamon	2 mL
½ tsp	vanilla	2 mL
3½ cups	water	875 mL
1 cup	apple juice	250 mL

1. In prepared slow cooker, combine steel-cut oats, wheat berries, apples, cinnamon and vanilla. Add water and apple juice. Cover and cook on High for 4 hours or on Low for 8 hours or overnight. Stir well.

Mindful Morsels

Breakfast is the most important meal of the day. Not only does a good breakfast help you feel energized and keep you productive throughout the day, it is also good for your heart and helps keep your weight under control. Research shows a link between eating breakfast, particularly whole grain cereals, and lower levels of cholesterol. For instance, a study in the *American Journal of Clinical Nutrition* reported that healthy women who skipped breakfast paid the price with higher levels of blood cholesterol and lower levels of insulin. They also snacked more during the day, consuming more calories than they would have if they had enjoyed a morning meal.

NUTRIENTS PER SERVING	
Calories	166
Fat	2.0 g
Saturates	0.4 g
Polyunsaturates	0.7 g
Monounsaturates	0.6 g
Cholesterol	0 mg
Sodium	7 mg
Carbohydrate	33.0 g
Fiber	4.4 g
Protein	4.9 g

AMERICA'S EXCHANGES	
1	Starch
1	Fruit

CANADA'S CHOICES	
2	Carbohydrate
½	Fat

MAKES 4 SERVINGS

Tips

If you are cooking this cereal in a large oval slow cooker, reduce the cooking time by half.

If you prefer a creamier version of this cereal, make it using half skim or 2% evaporated milk and half water. This will add 1 Low-fat Milk Exchange/ 1 Carbohydrate Choice per serving.

Irish Oatmeal

Although rolled oats are very tasty, my favorite oat cereal is steel-cut oats, which are often sold under the name "Irish Oatmeal." They have more flavor than rolled oats and an appealing crunchy texture.

- **Works best in a small (3½ quart) slow cooker (see Tips, left)**
- **Greased slow cooker stoneware**

1 cup	steel-cut oats	250 mL
½ tsp	salt	2 mL
4 cups	water	1 L

1. In prepared slow cooker, combine oats and salt. Add water. Cover and cook on High for 4 hours or on Low for 8 hours or overnight. Stir well.

Mindful Morsels

Many people enjoy a cup of coffee at breakfast and at other times throughout the day. In common with soft drinks, tea and chocolate, coffee contains caffeine. Experts recommend that healthy adults consume no more than 400 mg to 450 mg of caffeine per day, the amount in approximately three 8-oz (250 mL) cups of coffee. (Pregnant women should consume no more than 300 mg per day.) In addition to the well-known ability of too much caffeine to make you jittery, it can also affect bone density and risk of fractures. Studies indicate that people who drink coffee are less prone to these effects if they have enough calcium in their diet.

NUTRIENTS PER SERVING	
Calories	90
Fat	1.5 g
Saturates	0.4 g
Polyunsaturates	0.6 g
Monounsaturates	0.5 g
Cholesterol	0 mg
Sodium	296 mg
Carbohydrate	15.8 g
Fiber	2.1 g
Protein	3.6 g

AMERICA'S EXCHANGES	CANADA'S CHOICES
1 Starch	1 Carbohydrate

MAKES 8 SERVINGS

Tips

If you are cooking this cereal in a large oval slow cooker, reduce the cooking time by half.

Use plain or vanilla-flavored rice milk. Vary the quantity to suit your preference. Three cups (750 mL) produces a firmer result. If you like your cereal to be creamy, use the larger quantity.

Variation

Use half millet and half short-grain brown rice.

Creamy Morning Millet with Apples

If you're tired of the same old breakfast, perk up your taste buds by enjoying millet as a cereal. You can refrigerate leftovers for up to two days and reheat portions in the microwave.

- **Works best in a small (3½ quart) slow cooker (see Tips, left)**
- **Greased slow cooker stoneware**

1 cup	millet (see Tips, page 21)	250 mL
3 to 4 cups	enriched rice milk (see Tips, left)	750 mL to 1 L
3	apples, peeled, cored and chopped	3
¼ tsp	salt	1 mL

1. In prepared slow cooker stoneware, combine millet, rice milk, apples and salt. Cover and cook on High for 4 hours or on Low for 8 hours or overnight. Stir well and spoon into bowls.

NUTRIENTS PER SERVING	
Calories	171
Fat	1.7 g
Saturates	0.2 g
Polyunsaturates	0.6 g
Monounsaturates	0.8 g
Cholesterol	0 mg
Sodium	104 mg
Carbohydrate	36.1 g
Fiber	4.6 g
Protein	3.2 g

AMERICA'S EXCHANGES	
1½	Starch
1	Other Carbohydrate

CANADA'S CHOICES	
2	Carbohydrate

MAKES 10 SERVINGS

Tips

If you are cooking this cereal in a large oval slow cooker, reduce the cooking time by half.

Made with this quantity of liquid, the rice will be a bit crunchy around the edges. If you prefer a softer version or will be cooking it longer than 8 hours, add ½ cup (125 mL) of water or rice milk to the recipe.

Variation

Use half rice and half wheat berries.

Breakfast Rice

Simple yet delicious, this tasty combination couldn't be easier to make.

- **Works best in a small (3½ quart) slow cooker (see Tips, left)**
- **Greased slow cooker stoneware**

1 cup	brown rice	250 mL
4 cups	vanilla-flavored enriched rice milk	1 L
½ cup	dried cherries or cranberries	125 mL

1. In prepared slow cooker stoneware, combine rice, rice milk and cherries. Place a clean tea towel folded in half (so you will have two layers) over top of stoneware to absorb moisture. Cover and cook on High for 4 hours or on Low for up to 8 hours or overnight. Stir well and serve.

Mindful Morsels

Few foods are more ubiquitous than rice, which is eaten around the world. Although many people consume white rice, brown rice is far more nutritious. A complex carbohydrate, it contains much more fiber than white rice, as well as B vitamins and minerals such as manganese, selenium and magnesium. Because it also contains essential oils, which become rancid at room temperature, brown rice should be stored in the refrigerator in an airtight container.

NUTRIENTS PER SERVING	
Calories	145
Fat	1.5 g
Saturates	0.1 g
Polyunsaturates	0.4 g
Monounsaturates	0.9 g
Cholesterol	0 mg
Sodium	37 mg
Carbohydrate	30.9 g
Fiber	2.6 g
Protein	2.3 g

AMERICA'S EXCHANGES	
1	Starch
½	Fruit
½	Other Carbohydrate

CANADA'S CHOICES	
2	Carbohydrate

**MAKES 1 LOAF
(8 SLICES)**

Tips

This bread, like the others in this book, can be made in almost any kind of baking dish that will fit into your slow cooker. I have a variety of baking pans that work well: a small loaf pan (about 8 by 4 inches/20 by 10 cm) makes a traditionally shaped bread; a round (6 cup/1.5 L) soufflé dish or a square (7 inch/17.5 cm) baking dish produces slices of different shapes. All taste equally good.

Whole wheat flour quickly becomes rancid at room temperature and should be stored in the freezer. It will keep for up to a year and can be used directly from the freezer.

Whole Wheat Soda Bread

This homey bread is easy to make and is a delicious accompaniment to many main course dishes.

- **Large (minimum 5 quart) oval slow cooker**
- **Lightly greased 8- by 4-inch (20 by 10 cm) approx. loaf pan or 6 cup (1.5 L) soufflé or baking dish (see Tips, left)**

1 cup	whole wheat flour (see Tips, left)	250 mL
1 cup	all-purpose flour	250 mL
¾ tsp	baking soda	4 mL
¾ tsp	salt	4 mL
1¼ cups	buttermilk	300 mL

1. In a large bowl, mix together whole wheat and all-purpose flours, baking soda and salt. Make a well in the center, pour buttermilk into well and mix just until blended; do not overmix. Spread into prepared pan.

2. Cover pan tightly with foil and secure with string. Place pan in slow cooker stoneware and pour in enough boiling water to come 1 inch (2.5 cm) up the sides of the dish. Cover and cook on High for $2\frac{1}{2}$ to 3 hours, until bread springs back when touched lightly in the center. Unmold and serve warm.

Mindful Morsels

Substituting whole wheat flour for some or all of the white flour in any recipe is a healthful strategy. Unlike all-purpose flour, whole wheat flour includes all three nutrient-rich parts of the wheat berry: the bran, the germ and the endosperm. (White flour uses only the endosperm.) Whole wheat flour has more protein, fiber, niacin, pantothenic acid and vitamins E and B_6 than white flour. It is also much higher in magnesium and zinc. The fiber in whole wheat flour is one of its most valuable attributes.

NUTRIENTS PER SLICE	
Calories	123
Fat	0.8 g
Saturates	0.3 g
Polyunsaturates	0.2 g
Monounsaturates	0.2 g
Cholesterol	1 mg
Sodium	379 mg
Carbohydrate	24.7 g
Fiber	2.3 g
Protein	4.9 g

AMERICA'S EXCHANGES	
1½	Starch

CANADA'S CHOICES	
1½	Carbohydrate

MAKES 1 LOAF (8 SLICES)

Caraway Soda Bread

I love the caraway flavor in this classic Irish soda bread. It makes a great accompaniment to hearty soups and stews.

Tips

This bread, like the others in this book, can be made in almost any kind of baking dish that will fit into your slow cooker. I have a variety of baking pans that work well: a small loaf pan (about 8 by 4 inches/20 by 10 cm) makes a traditionally shaped bread; a round (6 cup/1.5 L) soufflé dish or a square (7 inch/17.5 cm) baking dish produces slices of different shapes. All taste equally good.

If you don't like the texture of whole caraway seeds, toast them in a dry skillet over medium heat, stirring, until fragrant, about 3 minutes, then grind them in a mortar or a spice grinder before adding to the dry ingredients.

- **Large (minimum 5 quart) oval slow cooker**
- **Lightly greased 8- by 4-inch (20 by 10 cm) approx. loaf pan or 6 cup (1.5 L) soufflé or baking dish (see Tips, left)**

1 cup	whole wheat flour	250 mL
1 cup	all-purpose flour, unbleached if possible	250 mL
2 tsp	caraway seeds (see Tips, left)	10 mL
2 tsp	granulated sugar	10 mL
1 tsp	baking soda	5 mL
½ tsp	salt	2 mL
¾ cup	buttermilk	175 mL
2 tbsp	olive oil	25 mL

1. In a large bowl, mix together whole wheat and all-purpose flours, caraway seeds, sugar, baking soda and salt. Make a well in the center.

2. In measuring cup, stir together buttermilk and olive oil. Pour into well and mix just until blended; do not overmix. Knead several times to make dough fit the shape of your pan and place in prepared pan.

3. Cover pan tightly with aluminum foil. Place in slow cooker stoneware and pour in enough boiling water to come 1 inch (2.5 cm) up the sides of the dish. Cover and cook on High for 2½ to 3 hours, until bread springs back when touched lightly in the center. Unmold and serve warm.

NUTRIENTS PER SLICE	
Calories	153
Fat	4.1 g
Saturates	0.7 g
Polyunsaturates	0.5 g
Monounsaturates	2.6 g
Cholesterol	1 mg
Sodium	315 mg
Carbohydrate	25.2 g
Fiber	2.4 g
Protein	4.5 g

AMERICA'S EXCHANGES	
1½	Starch
½	Fat

CANADA'S CHOICES	
1½	Carbohydrate
1	Fat

**MAKES 1 LOAF
(10 SLICES)**

Tips

This bread, like the others in this book, can be made in almost any kind of baking dish that will fit into your slow cooker. I have a variety of baking pans that work well: a small loaf pan (about 8 by 4 inches/20 by 10 cm) makes a traditionally shaped bread; a round (6 cup/1.5 L) soufflé dish or a square (7 inch/17.5 cm) baking dish produces slices of different shapes. All taste equally good.

To ease cleanup, mix the dry ingredients on a sheet of waxed paper, instead of using a bowl.

Banana Walnut Oat Bread

Serve this moist and flavorful bread as a dessert or for a breakfast on the run.

- **Large (minimum 5 quart) oval slow cooker**
- **Greased 8- by 4-inch (20 by 10 cm) approx. loaf pan or 6 cup (1.5 L) soufflé or baking dish (see Tips, left)**

⅓ cup	butter, softened	75 mL
⅔ cup	brown sugar	150 mL
2	eggs	2
3	ripe bananas, mashed (about 1¼ cups/300 mL)	3
¾ cup	all-purpose flour, unbleached if possible	175 mL
¾ cup	rolled oats (not quick-cooking)	175 mL
2 tbsp	milled flaxseeds	25 mL
2 tsp	baking powder	10 mL
½ tsp	salt	2 mL
¼ tsp	baking soda	1 mL
½ cup	finely chopped walnuts	125 mL

1. In a bowl, beat butter and sugar until light and creamy. Add eggs, one at a time, beating until incorporated. Beat in bananas.

2. In a separate bowl (see Tips, left), combine flour, oats, flaxseeds, baking powder, salt and baking soda. Add to banana mixture, stirring just until combined; do not overmix. Fold in walnuts.

3. Spoon batter into prepared pan. Cover tightly with foil and secure with a string. Place pan in slow cooker stoneware and pour in enough boiling water to come 1 inch (2.5 cm) up the sides. Cover and cook on High for 3 hours, until a tester inserted in the center comes out clean. Unmold and serve warm or let cool.

NUTRIENTS PER SLICE	
Calories	262
Fat	12.2 g
Saturates	4.7 g
Polyunsaturates	3.8 g
Monounsaturates	3.0 g
Cholesterol	57 mg
Sodium	278 mg
Carbohydrate	35.3 g
Fiber	2.4 g
Protein	4.8 g

AMERICA'S EXCHANGES	
1½	Starch
½	Fruit
½	Other Carbohydrate
2	Fat

CANADA'S CHOICES	
2	Carbohydrate
2	Fat

**MAKES 1 LOAF
(12 HALF-SLICES)**

Tips

This bread, like the others in this book, can be made in almost any kind of baking dish that will fit into your slow cooker. I have a variety of baking pans that work well: a small loaf pan (about 8 by 4 inches/20 by 10 cm) makes a traditionally shaped bread; a round (6 cup/ 1.5 L) soufflé dish or a square (7 inch/17.5 cm) baking dish produces slices of different shapes. All taste equally good.

Whole wheat flour quickly becomes rancid at room temperature and should be stored in the freezer. It will keep for up to a year and can be used directly from the freezer.

Carrot Bread

Serve this tasty bread as a snack or for a healthy breakfast on the run.

- **Large (minimum 5 quart) oval slow cooker**
- **Greased 8- by 4-inch (20 by 10 cm) approx. loaf pan or 6 cup (1.5 L) soufflé or baking dish (see Tips, left)**

1½ cups	all-purpose flour	375 mL
½ cup	whole wheat flour (see Tips, left)	125 mL
2 tsp	baking powder	10 mL
1 tsp	ground cinnamon	5 mL
½ tsp	ground cloves	2 mL
½ tsp	salt	2 mL
½ cup	packed brown sugar	125 mL
¼ cup	granulated sugar	50 mL
3 tbsp	olive oil	45 mL
1	egg, beaten	1
¾ cup	low-fat plain yogurt	175 mL
1½ cups	shredded peeled carrots	375 mL
⅓ cup	chopped pecans	75 mL

1. In a bowl, combine all-purpose and whole wheat flours, baking powder, cinnamon, cloves and salt.

2. In a separate bowl, beat together brown and granulated sugars, olive oil, egg and yogurt. Add to flour mixture, stirring just until combined; do not overmix. Fold in carrots and pecans.

3. Spoon batter into prepared pan. Cover tightly with foil and secure with a string. Place pan in slow cooker stoneware and pour in enough boiling water to come 1 inch (2.5 cm) up the sides of the dish. Cover and cook on High for 4 hours, until a tester inserted in the center of the loaf comes out clean. Unmold and serve warm or let cool. Cut into 6 thick slices, then cut each slice in half.

NUTRIENTS PER HALF-SLICE	
Calories	199
Fat	6.5 g
Saturates	0.9 g
Polyunsaturates	1.0 g
Monounsaturates	4.1 g
Cholesterol	16 mg
Sodium	169 mg
Carbohydrate	32.1 g
Fiber	1.7 g
Protein	4.0 g

AMERICA'S EXCHANGES	
1	Starch
1	Other Carbohydrate
1	Fat

CANADA'S CHOICES	
2	Carbohydrate
1½	Fat

**MAKES 1 LOAF
(10 SLICES)**

Tips

This bread, like the others in this book, can be made in almost any kind of baking dish that will fit into your slow cooker. I have a variety of baking pans that work well: a small loaf pan (about 8 by 4 inches/20 by 10 cm) makes a traditionally shaped bread; a round (6 cup/ 1.5 L) soufflé dish or a square (7 inch/17.5 cm) baking dish produces slices of different shapes. All taste equally good.

If you prefer smaller round loaves, make this bread using three 19 oz (540 mL) vegetable tins, washed dried and sprayed with olive oil. Cover tops tightly with foil and reduce cooking time to 2 hours.

I like to use less-processed sugars, such as muscovado or evaporated cane juice sugar (Sucanat™ or Rapadura™).

Pumpkin Date Loaf

Everyone loves this moist and dense loaf. Refrigerate any leftovers and serve them cold or, if you prefer, reheated in the microwave.

- **Large (minimum 5 quart) oval slow cooker**
- **Greased 8- by 4-inch (20 by 10 cm) approx. loaf pan or 6 cup (1.5 L) soufflé or baking dish (see Tips, left)**

1 cup	all-purpose flour, unbleached if possible	250 mL
1 tsp	baking soda	5 mL
½ tsp	salt	2 mL
½ cup	finely chopped pitted soft dates, such as Medjool (5 to 6 dates)	125 mL
½ cup	finely chopped pecans	125 mL
2	eggs	2
½ cup	packed muscovado or evaporated cane juice sugar	125 mL
2 tbsp	olive oil	25 mL
1 cup	pumpkin purée (not pie filling)	250 mL
1 tsp	ground cinnamon	5 mL
½ tsp	freshly grated nutmeg	2 mL
¼ tsp	ground ginger	1 mL

1. In a large bowl, mix together flour, baking soda and salt. Add dates and, using your fingers, separate any pieces of dates that are stuck together, ensuring that the bits are coated in flour. Add pecans and stir to blend. Make a well in the center.

2. In a separate bowl, beat eggs, sugar and olive oil until smooth and blended. Add pumpkin, cinnamon, nutmeg and ginger and mix well. Add to well in dry ingredients and mix just until blended; do not overmix.

3. Spoon batter into prepared pan. Cover tightly with foil and secure with a string. Place pan in slow cooker stoneware and pour in enough boiling water to come 1 inch (2.5 cm) up the sides. Cover and cook on High for 3 hours, until a tester inserted in the center of the loaf comes out clean. Unmold and serve warm or let cool.

NUTRIENTS PER SLICE	
Calories	200
Fat	8.2 g
Saturates	1.1 g
Polyunsaturates	1.7 g
Monounsaturates	4.8 g
Cholesterol	38 mg
Sodium	250 mg
Carbohydrate	30.0 g
Fiber	2.3 g
Protein	3.5 g

AMERICA'S EXCHANGES	
1	Starch
1	Other Carbohydrate
1½	Fat

CANADA'S CHOICES	
2	Carbohydrate
1½	Fat

Black Bean and Salsa Dip

**MAKES ABOUT
3 CUPS (750 ML)**

(1/4 cup/50 mL per serving)

Tips

If you use a five-alarm salsa in this dip, you may find it too spicy with the addition of jalapeño pepper.

To toast cumin seeds: Place seeds in a dry skillet over medium heat, stirring, until fragrant, about 3 minutes. Immediately transfer to a mortar or a spice grinder and grind. If you prefer to use ground cumin, substitute half of the quantity called for.

For a smoother dip, purée the beans in a food processor or mash with a potato masher before adding to stoneware.

This tasty, Cuban-inspired dip is a welcome treat any time of the day. Serve with tortilla chips, tostadas or crisp crackers (remember to count the America's Exchanges/Canada's Choices they contribute), or with fresh vegetables cut for dipping (crudités), a Free Food/Extra.

* **Works best in a small (maximum 3 1/2 quart) slow cooker**

1	can (19 oz/540 mL) canned black beans, drained and rinsed, or 2 cups (500 mL) cooked dried black beans (see Variation, page 231)	1
1	package (8 oz/250 g) light cream cheese, cubed	1
1/2 cup	tomato salsa	125 mL
1/4 cup	light sour cream	50 mL
2 tsp	cumin seeds, toasted and ground (see Tips, left)	10 mL
1 tsp	chili powder	5 mL
1 tsp	cracked black peppercorns	5 mL
1	jalapeño pepper, finely chopped, optional (see Tips, left)	1
	Finely chopped green onion, optional	
	Finely chopped cilantro, optional	

1. In slow cooker stoneware, combine beans, cream cheese, salsa, sour cream, toasted cumin, chili powder, peppercorns and jalapeño pepper, if using. Cover and cook on High for 1 hour. Stir again and cook on High for an additional 30 minutes, until mixture is hot and bubbly. Serve immediately or set temperature at Low until ready to serve. Garnish with green onion and/or cilantro, if desired.

> ### Mindful Morsels
>
> Look for low-fat baked varieties of "dippers" (no more than 3 g of fat per 50 g) and estimate the weight of one piece from the Nutrition Facts on the package. Twenty grams of low-fat baked tortilla chips is equivalent to a Starch Exchange/ Carbohydrate Choice. Because they are usually high in sodium, dippers should be consumed in small quantities.

NUTRIENTS PER SERVING	
Calories	42
Fat	1.9 g
Saturates	0 g
Polyunsaturates	0.1 g
Monounsaturates	0 g
Cholesterol	0 mg
Sodium	145 mg
Carbohydrate	9.1 g
Fiber	2.3 g
Protein	4.2 g

AMERICA'S EXCHANGES	
1/2	Starch
1/2	Lean Meat

CANADA'S CHOICES	
1/2	Carbohydrate
1/2	Meat and Alternatives

**MAKES ABOUT
3½ CUPS (875 ML)**
(¼ cup/50 mL per serving)

Tip

If you are using fresh spinach leaves in this recipe, take care to wash them thoroughly, as they can be quite gritty. To wash spinach: Fill a clean sink with lukewarm water. Remove the tough stems and submerge the tender leaves in the water, swishing to remove the grit. Rinse thoroughly in a colander under cold running water, checking carefully to ensure that no sand remains. If you are using frozen spinach in this recipe, thaw and squeeze the excess moisture out before adding to the slow cooker. Dry thoroughly before adding to the slow cooker. If excess moisture is not removed from the dip, it will be quite runny — but still delicious!

Spicy Spinach Dip

Here's a great dip with a bit of punch. If you are a heat seeker, add the extra jalapeño pepper and use extra hot salsa.

- **Works best in a small (maximum 3½ quart) slow cooker**

1 lb	fresh spinach, stems removed, or 1 package (10 oz/300 g) spinach leaves, thawed if frozen (see Tip, left)	500 g
2 cups	shredded light Monterey Jack cheese	500 mL
½ cup	tomato salsa	125 mL
¼ cup	light sour cream	50 mL
4	green onions, white part only, finely chopped	4
1 to 2	jalapeño peppers, seeds removed and finely chopped	1 to 2
¼ tsp	freshly ground black pepper	1 mL
	Low-fat baked tostadas or tortilla chips	

1. In slow cooker stoneware, combine spinach, cheese, salsa, sour cream, green onions, jalapeño peppers and black pepper. Cover and cook on High for 2 hours, until hot and bubbly. Stir well and serve with tostadas or tortilla chips.

> ### Mindful Morsels
>
> The colorful vegetables in this dip make it more than just pretty to look at. A healthy diet containing generous amounts of vegetables may help reduce the risk of some types of cancer. This protective effect appears to be related to brightly colored pigments, such as beta carotene and lycopene, and their interactions with other components of the foods we eat.

NUTRIENTS PER SERVING	
Calories	66
Fat	3.8 g
Saturates	2.3 g
Polyunsaturates	0.2 g
Monounsaturates	0.9 g
Cholesterol	10 mg
Sodium	153 mg
Carbohydrate	2.4 g
Fiber	1 g
Protein	5.9 g

AMERICA'S EXCHANGES	
1	Lean Meat
1	Free Food

CANADA'S CHOICES	
1	Meat and Alternatives
1	Extra

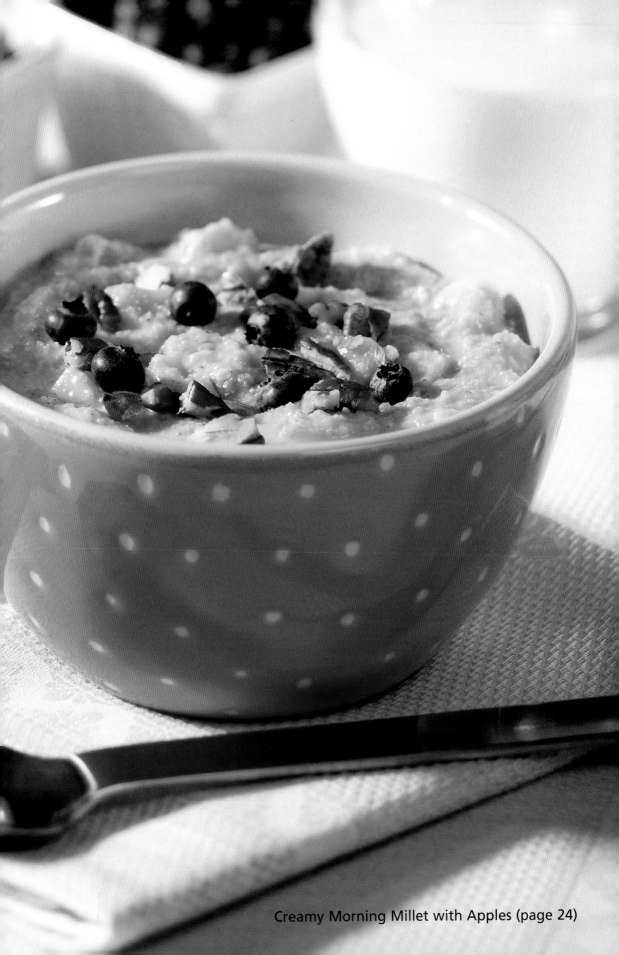

Creamy Morning Millet with Apples (page 24)

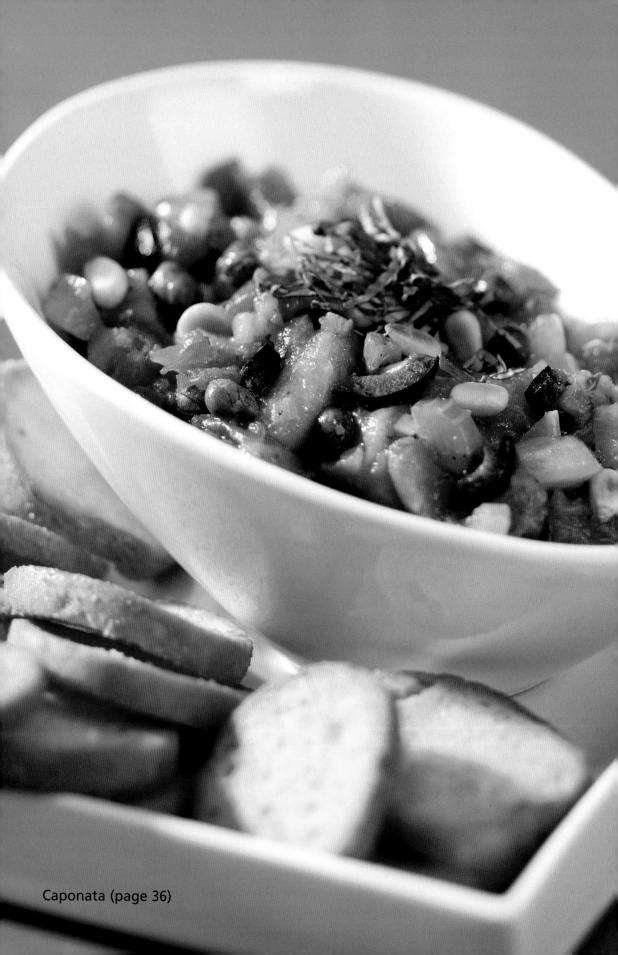

Caponata (page 36)

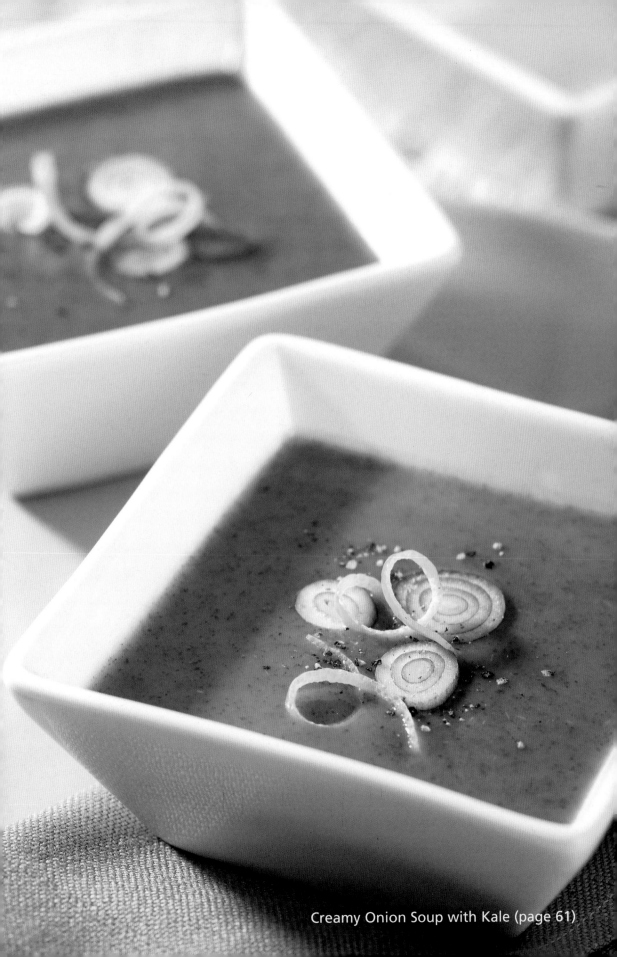

Creamy Onion Soup with Kale (page 61)

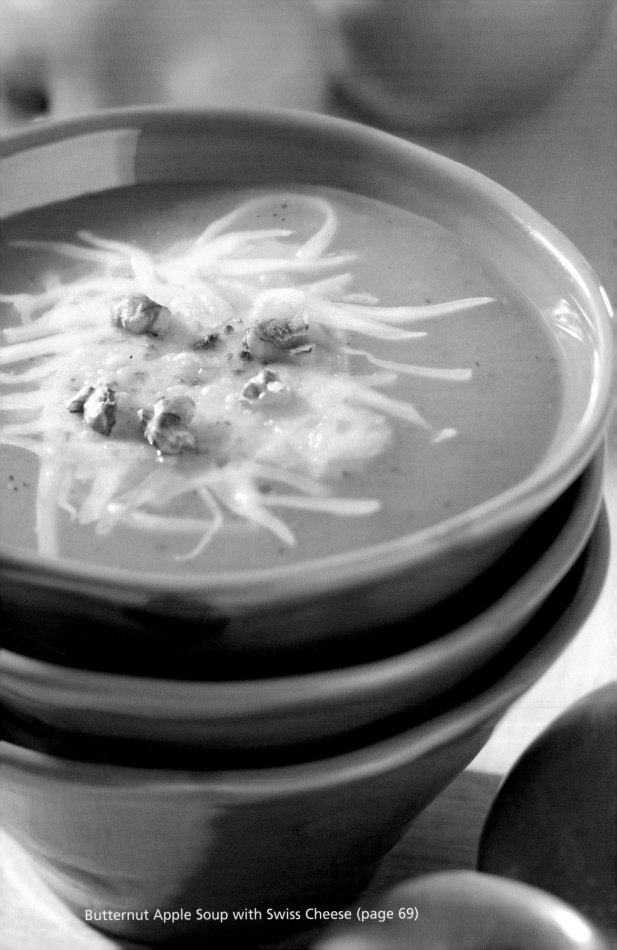

Butternut Apple Soup with Swiss Cheese (page 69)

Sumptuous Spinach and Artichoke Dip

MAKES ABOUT 4 CUPS (1 L)
(⅓ cup/75 mL per serving)

This classic dip has its roots in Provençal cuisine, where vegetables are baked with cheese and served as a gratin. Serve with crudités (bite-size vegetable dippers) — a Free Food/Extra — or with low-fat baked tortilla chips (remember to count them as part of your America's Exchanges/Canada's Choices).

Tips

If you are using fresh spinach leaves in this recipe, take care to wash them thoroughly, as they can be quite gritty. To wash spinach: Fill a clean sink with lukewarm water. Remove the tough stems and submerge the tender leaves in the water, swishing to remove the grit. Rinse thoroughly in a colander under cold running water, checking carefully to ensure that no sand remains. If you are using frozen spinach in this recipe, thaw and squeeze the excess moisture out before adding to the slow cooker.

If you prefer a smoother dip, place spinach and artichokes in a food processor, in separate batches, and pulse until desired degree of fineness is achieved. Then combine with remaining ingredients in slow cooker stoneware.

- **Works best in a small (maximum 3½ quart) slow cooker**

1 cup	shredded part-skim mozzarella cheese	250 mL
8 oz	light cream cheese, cubed	250 g
¼ cup	freshly grated Parmesan cheese	50 mL
1	clove garlic, minced	1
¼ tsp	freshly ground black pepper	1 mL
1	can (14 oz/398 mL) artichokes, drained and finely chopped	1
1 lb	fresh spinach, stems removed, or 1 package (10 oz/300 g) spinach leaves, thawed if frozen (see Tips, left)	500 g

1. In slow cooker stoneware, combine cheese, cream cheese, Parmesan, garlic, pepper, artichokes and spinach. Cover and cook on High for 2 hours, until hot and bubbly. Stir well.

Mindful Morsels

One-half cup (125 mL) of cooked spinach or other dark green leafy vegetable is an excellent source of folacin, a B vitamin that is required for the proper development of all cells in the body.

NUTRIENTS PER SERVING	
Calories	97
Fat	6.1 g
Saturates	3.6 g
Polyunsaturates	0.2 g
Monounsaturates	1.8 g
Cholesterol	20 mg
Sodium	311 mg
Carbohydrate	4.7 g
Fiber	2.0 g
Protein	6.8 g

AMERICA'S EXCHANGES	
1	Vegetable
½	High-fat Meat

CANADA'S CHOICES	
1	Meat and Alternatives
1	Extra

**MAKES ABOUT
2 CUPS (500 ML)**
(2 tbsp/25 mL per serving)

Tip

To toast pine nuts: Place pine nuts in a dry skillet over medium heat. Cook, stirring constantly, until they begin to turn light gold, 3 to 4 minutes. Remove from heat and immediately transfer to a small bowl. Once they begin to brown, they can burn very quickly.

Artichoke, Sun-Dried Tomato and Goat Cheese Spread

Serve this sophisticated spread on leaves of Belgian endive. Or spoon it into a pottery bowl and surround with pieces of flatbread (be sure to count it in your America's Exchanges/Canada's Choices).

- **Works best in a small (maximum 3½ quart) slow cooker**

1	can (14 oz/398 mL) artichokes, drained and finely chopped	1
4	sun-dried tomatoes, packed in olive oil, drained and finely chopped	4
2	cloves garlic, crushed	2
¼ tsp	salt	1 mL
¼ tsp	freshly ground black pepper	1 mL
8 oz	lower-fat goat cheese, crumbled	250 g
	Belgian endive, optional	
¼ cup	toasted pine nuts, optional	50 mL

1. In slow cooker stoneware, combine artichokes, sun-dried tomatoes, garlic, salt and pepper. Cover and cook on High for 1 hour.

2. Add goat cheese and stir to combine. Cover and cook on High for 1 hour, until hot and bubbly. Stir well. Spoon into a bowl or spread on leaves of Belgian endive and top with toasted pine nuts, if using.

NUTRIENTS PER SERVING	
Calories	49
Fat	3.1 g
Saturates	2.1 g
Polyunsaturates	0.1 g
Monounsaturates	0.8 g
Cholesterol	7 mg
Sodium	148 mg
Carbohydrate	2.4 g
Fiber	1 g
Protein	3.3 g

AMERICA'S EXCHANGES	CANADA'S CHOICES
½ High-fat Meat	½ Meat and Alternatives

Chilly Dilly Eggplant

**MAKES ABOUT
4 CUPS (1 L)**
(¼ cup/50 mL per serving)

This is a versatile recipe, delicious as a dip with raw vegetables or on pita triangles, as well as a sandwich spread on crusty French bread. It also makes a wonderful addition to a mezes or tapas-style meal. Although it is tasty warm, the flavor dramatically improves if it is thoroughly chilled before serving.

Tip

Although eggplant is delicious when properly cooked, some varieties tend to be bitter. Since the bitterness is concentrated under the skin, I peel eggplant before using. Sprinkling the pieces with salt and leaving them to "sweat" for an hour or two also draws out the bitter juice. If time is short, blanch the pieces for a minute or two in heavily salted water. In either case, rinse thoroughly in fresh cold water and, using your hands, squeeze out the excess moisture. Pat dry with paper towels and it's ready for cooking.

• **Works best in a small (maximum 3½ quart) slow cooker**

3 tbsp	olive oil	45 mL
2	large eggplants, peeled, cut into 1-inch (2.5 cm) cubes and drained of excess moisture (see Tip, left)	2
2	onions, chopped	2
4	cloves garlic, chopped	4
1 tsp	dried oregano leaves	5 mL
1 tsp	salt	5 mL
½ tsp	freshly ground black pepper	2 mL
1 tbsp	balsamic or red wine vinegar	15 mL
½ cup	chopped fresh dill	125 mL
	Dill sprigs, optional	

1. In a skillet, heat 2 tbsp (25 mL) of the oil over medium-high heat for 30 seconds. Add eggplant, in batches, and cook, stirring and tossing, until it begins to brown, about 3 minutes per batch. Transfer to slow cooker stoneware.

2. Reduce heat to medium. Add more oil, if necessary, and cook onions, stirring, until softened, about 3 minutes. Add garlic, oregano, salt and pepper and cook, stirring, for 1 minute. Transfer to slow cooker stoneware and stir to combine thoroughly. Cover and cook on Low for 7 to 8 hours or on High for 4 hours, until eggplant is tender.

3. Transfer contents of slow cooker (in batches, if necessary) to a blender or food processor. Add vinegar and dill and process until smooth, scraping down sides of bowl at halfway point. Taste for seasoning and adjust. Spoon into a small serving bowl and chill thoroughly. Garnish with sprigs of dill, if using.

Make Ahead

You'll achieve the best results if you make this a day ahead and chill thoroughly before serving, or cook overnight, purée in the morning and chill.

NUTRIENTS PER SERVING	
Calories	47
Fat	2.7 g
Saturates	0.4 g
Polyunsaturates	0.3 g
Monounsaturates	1.9 g
Cholesterol	0 mg
Sodium	148 mg
Carbohydrate	5.9 g
Fiber	1.8 g
Protein	0.8 g

AMERICA'S EXCHANGES	
1	Vegetable
½	Fat

CANADA'S CHOICES	
½	Fat
1	Extra

Caponata

(see Tip, page 35)

**MAKES ABOUT
4 CUPS (1 L)**

(¼ cup/50 mL per serving)

Tip

To cut the basil into chiffonade, stack the leaves, 4 at a time, roll them into a cigar shape and slice as thinly as you can.

Make ahead

You'll achieve the best results if you make the caponata a day ahead and chill overnight in the refrigerator.

This robust spread is a treat from Sicily. Serve it on crostini or with crackers, pita bread or crudités such as celery sticks. It keeps, covered, in the refrigerator for up to one week.

• **Works best in a small (maximum 3½ quart) slow cooker**

2 tbsp	balsamic vinegar	25 mL
1 tsp	packed brown sugar	5 mL
3 tbsp	olive oil	45 mL
1	medium eggplant, peeled, cut into 1-inch (2.5 cm) cubes and drained of excess moisture (see Tip, page 35)	1
1	onion, finely chopped	1
2	stalks celery, finely chopped	2
4	cloves garlic, minced	4
1 tsp	dried oregano leaves	5 mL
½ tsp	cracked black peppercorns	2 mL
1	can (14 oz/398 mL) diced tomatoes, including juice	1
½ cup	chopped pitted black olives	125 mL
1 tbsp	drained capers	15 mL
2 tbsp	toasted pine nuts (see Tip, page 34)	25 mL
2 tbsp	chiffonade of basil leaves, optional (see Tip, left)	25 mL

1. In a small bowl, combine vinegar and brown sugar. Stir until sugar dissolves. Set aside.

2. In a skillet, heat 2 tbsp (25 mL) of the oil over medium-high heat for 30 seconds. Add eggplant, in batches, and cook, stirring and tossing, until it begins to brown, about 3 minutes per batch. Transfer to slow cooker stoneware.

3. In same skillet over medium heat, adding more oil if necessary, cook onion and celery, stirring, until softened, about 5 minutes. Add garlic, oregano and peppercorns and cook, stirring, for 1 minute. Add tomatoes, with juice, and balsamic mixture and bring to a boil. Boil for 1 minute to reduce liquid. Transfer to stoneware and stir thoroughly.

4. Cover and cook on Low for 7 to 8 hours or on High for 4 hours, until eggplant is tender. Stir in olives and capers. Transfer to a serving bowl. Cover and refrigerate for 2 hours or overnight. Garnish with pine nuts and basil, if using.

NUTRIENTS PER SERVING	
Calories	54
Fat	3.6 g
Saturates	0.5 g
Polyunsaturates	0.5 g
Monounsaturates	2.4 g
Cholesterol	0 mg
Sodium	100 mg
Carbohydrate	5.3 g
Fiber	1.4 g
Protein	1.0 g

AMERICA'S EXCHANGES	
1	Vegetable
1	Fat

CANADA'S CHOICES	
1	Fat
1	Extra

Soups

Basic Vegetable Stock

MAKES ABOUT 12 CUPS (3 L)
(1 cup/250 mL per serving)

These stock recipes, each of which make enough for two average soup recipes, can be made ahead and frozen. For convenience, cook them overnight in the slow cooker. If your slow cooker is not large enough to make a full batch, you can halve the recipes.

* **Large (minimum 6 quart) slow cooker**

8	carrots, scrubbed and coarsely chopped	8
6	stalks celery, coarsely chopped	6
3	onions, coarsely chopped	3
3	cloves garlic, coarsely chopped	3
6	sprigs parsley	6
3	bay leaves	3
10	black peppercorns	10
1 tsp	dried thyme leaves	5 mL
12 cups	water	3 L

1. In slow cooker stoneware, combine carrots, celery, onions, garlic, parsley, bay leaves, peppercorns and water. Cover and cook on Low for 8 hours or on High for 4 hours. Strain and discard solids. Cover and refrigerate for up to 5 days or freeze in an airtight container.

Tip

To freeze stock, transfer to airtight containers in small, measured portions (2 cups/500 mL or 4 cups/1 L are handy), leaving at least 1-inch (2.5 cm) headspace for expansion. Refrigerate until chilled, cover and freeze for up to 3 months. Thaw in refrigerator or microwave before using.

Variation

Enhanced Vegetable Stock:
To enhance 8 cups (2 L) Basic Vegetable Stock, combine in a large saucepan over medium heat with 2 carrots, peeled and coarsely chopped, 1 tbsp (15 mL) tomato paste, 1 tsp (5 mL) celery seeds, 1 tsp (5 mL) cracked black peppercorns, 1/2 tsp (2 mL) dried thyme leaves, 4 parsley sprigs, 1 bay leaf and 1 cup (250 mL) white wine. Bring to a boil. Reduce heat to low and simmer, covered, for 30 minutes, then strain and discard solids.

Mindful Morsels

Basic Vegetable Stock contains virtually no nutrients, so it counts as a Free Food/Extra. The advantage to making your own vegetable broth is to reduce your consumption of sodium. One cup (250 mL) of this broth, with no salt added, contains 0 mg of sodium. The same quantity of a purchased broth will likely contain 500 to 800 mg of sodium.

NUTRIENTS PER SERVING	
Calories	10
Fat	0 g
Saturates	0 g
Polyunsaturates	0 g
Monounsaturates	0 g
Cholesterol	0 mg
Sodium	5 mg
Carbohydrate	2 g
Fiber	0 g
Protein	0 g

AMERICA'S EXCHANGES	
1	Free Food

CANADA'S CHOICES	
1	Extra

Tip

The more economical parts of the chicken, such as necks, backs and wings, make the best stock.

Homemade Chicken Stock

There's nothing quite like the flavor of homemade chicken stock. It's very easy to make — you can cook it overnight, strain it in the morning and refrigerate it during the day. By the time you return home, the fat will have congealed on top and you can skim it off.

- **Large (minimum 6 quart) slow cooker**

4 lbs	bone-in skin-on chicken parts (see Tip, left)	2 kg
3	onions, coarsely chopped	3
4	carrots, scrubbed and coarsely chopped	4
4	stalks celery, coarsely chopped	4
6	sprigs parsley	6
3	bay leaves	3
10	black peppercorns	10
1 tsp	dried thyme leaves	5 mL
12 cups	water	3 L

1. In slow cooker stoneware, combine chicken, onions, carrots, celery, parsley, bay leaves, peppercorns, thyme and water. Cover and cook on High for 8 hours. Strain into a large bowl, discarding solids. Refrigerate liquid until fat forms on surface, about 6 hours. Skim off fat. Cover and refrigerate for up to 5 days.

Stock and Broth

What's the difference between stock and broth? The answer depends a lot on who you ask. Generally speaking, stock is prepared by simmering meat, fish or poultry (often just the bones) and/or vegetables, together with seasonings, for several hours. The stock is then strained off. Broth may be the liquid in which meat has been cooked, the clear portion of a soup with other ingredients or a soup on its own, usually with added seasonings.

In this book, "lower-salt chicken broth" and "lower-salt vegetable broth" refer to commercially prepared products, in cans (usually condensed, which need to be diluted) or cartons (ready-to-use). Look for a product with less than 600 mg of sodium per cup (250 mL). Typically, they will be labeled "reduced-salt" or "reduced-sodium," but there are others that qualify. Use the sodium values on the Nutrition Facts panel to help you choose.

When Homemade Chicken Stock or Basic Vegetable Stock is called for, be sure to make it without salt.

NUTRIENTS PER SERVING	
Calories	21
Fat	1.1 g
Saturates	0.3 g
Polyunsaturates	0.2 g
Monounsaturates	0.4 g
Cholesterol	20 mg
Sodium	21 mg
Carbohydrate	0.1 g
Fiber	0.1 g
Protein	2.7 g

AMERICA'S EXCHANGES		CANADA'S CHOICES	
1	Free Food	1	Extra

Tip

Three-quarters of a cup (175 mL) of dried beans yields about 2 cups (500 mL) when cooked, equivalent to a 19-oz (540 mL) can of beans, drained and rinsed.

South American Black Bean Soup

This mouthwatering combination of black beans, lime juice and cilantro with just a hint of hot pepper is one of my favorite one-dish meals. To jack up the heat, add a chopped jalapeño along with the cayenne. The flavor of this soup actually improves if it is allowed to sit overnight and then reheated. Garnish with finely chopped cilantro, light sour cream or salsa. One tablespoon (15 mL) of light sour cream is 1 Free Food/Extra, as is ¼ cup (50 mL) salsa.

- **Works best in a large (minimum 5 quart) slow cooker**

6	slices bacon, chopped	6
1 tbsp	olive oil	15 mL
2	onions, finely chopped	2
2	stalks celery, finely chopped	2
2	carrots, peeled and finely chopped	2
2	cloves garlic, minced	2
2 tbsp	cumin seeds, toasted and ground (see Tip, page 31)	25 mL
1 tbsp	dried oregano leaves	15 mL
1 tsp	dried thyme leaves	5 mL
1 tsp	cracked black peppercorns	5 mL
2 tbsp	tomato paste	25 mL
6 cups	lower-salt chicken broth	1.5 L
4 cups	cooked dried or canned black beans, drained and rinsed (see Tip, left)	1 L
⅓ cup	freshly squeezed lime juice	75 mL
¼ tsp	cayenne pepper	1 mL
1	jalapeño pepper, chopped, optional	1

1. In a skillet, cook bacon over medium-high heat until crisp. Drain thoroughly on paper towel. Cover and refrigerate until ready to use. Drain fat from pan. Add oil.

2. Reduce heat to medium. Add onions, celery and carrots and cook, stirring, until vegetables are softened, about 7 minutes. Add garlic, toasted cumin, oregano, thyme and peppercorns and cook, stirring, for 1 minute. Add tomato paste and stir to combine thoroughly. Transfer to stoneware. Stir in broth.

NUTRIENTS PER SERVING	
Calories	141
Fat	4.9 g
Saturates	1.2 g
Polyunsaturates	0.7 g
Monounsaturates	2.5 g
Cholesterol	4 mg
Sodium	614 mg
Carbohydrate	17.8 g
Fiber	5.2 g
Protein	7.9 g

AMERICA'S EXCHANGES	
1	Vegetable
2	Lean Meat

CANADA'S CHOICES	
1	Carbohydrate
½	Meat and Alternatives
½	Fat

Make Ahead

This soup can be partially prepared before it is cooked. Complete Steps 1 and 2. Cover and refrigerate for up to 2 days. When you're ready to cook, continue with the recipe.

3. Add beans and reserved bacon and stir well. Cover and cook on Low for 8 to 10 hours or on High for 4 to 6 hours, until vegetables are tender. Stir in lime juice, cayenne and jalapeño, if using. Cover and cook on High for 10 minutes, until heated through. Working in batches, purée soup in a food processor or blender. (You can also do this in the stoneware using an immersion blender.) Spoon into bowls and garnish.

Mindful Morsels

Dried legumes, such as black beans, kidney beans, lentils and split peas, are very nutritious. They provide not only protein, but also slowly released carbohydrate that causes a smaller increase in blood glucose than many other carbohydrate-containing foods. Half a cup (125 mL) of cooked beans contains about 7 g of protein (and typically, less than 1 g of fat), making it a good alternative to meat, and is very high in fiber and folacin (a B vitamin). It also supplies thiamine and niacin and six minerals, including iron, magnesium, zinc and manganese, and has virtually no sodium when prepared without salt. Fiber-rich foods are also more filling and lengthen the time until you next feel hungry.

MAKES 8 SERVINGS

Tips

If your market is out of fennel, use 6 stalks of diced celery instead.

To toast fennel seeds: Place in a dry skillet over medium heat and cook, stirring, until seeds are fragrant, about 3 minutes. Immediately transfer to a mortar or a spice grinder and grind.

Adding the green beans while they are still frozen ensures that they will not be mushy when the soup has finished cooking. If you prefer to use fresh green beans, cut them into 2-inch (5 cm) lengths and cook them in a pot of boiling salted water for 4 minutes, until tender-crisp. Add them to the slow cooker after stirring in the paprika.

Two-Bean Soup with Pistou

I love the flavors in this classic French country soup: the hint of licorice in the fennel and the nip of paprika is nicely balanced by the pleasing blandness of the potatoes and beans.

- **Large (minimum 6 quart) slow cooker**

1 tbsp	olive oil	15 mL
3	onions, finely chopped	3
2	carrots, peeled and diced	2
1	bulb fennel, base and leafy stems discarded, bulb thinly sliced on the vertical and cut into ½-inch (1 cm) lengths (see Tips, left)	1
1 tsp	fennel seeds, toasted (see Tips, left)	5 mL
1	can (28 oz/796) diced tomatoes, including juice	1
6 cups	Basic Vegetable Stock or Homemade Chicken Stock (see recipes, pages 38 and 39) or lower-salt broth	1.5 L
2	potatoes, peeled and shredded	2
2	cans (each 14 oz/398 mL) white beans, drained and rinsed, or 2 cups (500 mL) dried white beans, soaked, cooked and drained (see Basic Beans, page 231)	2
2 cups	frozen sliced green beans (see Tips, left)	500 mL
2 tsp	paprika, dissolved in 1 tbsp (15 mL) water	10 mL
	Freshly ground black pepper	

Pistou

1 cup	packed fresh basil leaves	250 mL
4	cloves garlic, minced	4
½ cup	finely grated Parmesan cheese	125 mL
¼ cup	extra virgin olive oil	50 mL

1. In a skillet, heat oil over medium heat for 30 seconds. Add onions, carrots and fennel bulb and cook, stirring, until vegetables are softened, about 7 minutes. Add toasted fennel seeds and cook, stirring, for 1 minute. Add tomatoes with juice and bring to a boil. Transfer to slow cooker stoneware.

NUTRIENTS PER SERVING

Calories	270
Fat	11.1 g
Saturates	2.4 g
Polyunsaturates	1.1 g
Monounsaturates	6.8 g
Cholesterol	5 mg
Sodium	549 mg
Carbohydrate	35.2 g
Fiber	10.0 g
Protein	10.4 g

AMERICA'S EXCHANGES	
2	Starch
1	Lean Meat
1	Fat

CANADA'S CHOICES	
1½	Carbohydrate
1	Meat and Alternatives
1	Fat

You can partially prepare this soup ahead of time. Complete Step 1. Cover and refrigerate overnight or for up to 2 days. When you're ready to cook, continue with Steps 2 and 3.

2. Add stock, potatoes, white beans and green beans. Cover and cook on Low for 8 hours or on High for 4 hours, until vegetables are tender. Stir in paprika solution and season to taste with pepper. Cover and cook on High for 20 minutes.

3. **Pistou:** In a food processor fitted with a metal blade, combine basil, garlic and Parmesan. Process until smooth. Slowly add olive oil down the feeder tube until integrated. Ladle soup into bowls and top each serving with a dollop of pistou.

Mindful Morsels

Canned beans are high in sodium. In this recipe, they contribute about 250 mg of sodium per serving. You may want to look for reduced-sodium varieties or those with no salt added, or cook your own with no added salt. (See Basic Beans, page 231.) Rinsing also helps reduce the salt content.

MAKES 8 SERVINGS

Tip

If you can't find Swiss chard, use an equal quantity of spinach. Be sure to wash Swiss chard thoroughly like spinach (see Tip, page 32).

Ribollita

Originally intended as a method for using up leftover minestrone — hence the name ribollita, which means "twice cooked" — this hearty Italian soup has acquired an illustrious reputation of its own. The distinguishing ingredient is country-style bread, which is added to the soup and cooked in the broth. Drizzled with olive oil and sprinkled with grated Parmesan cheese, this makes a satisfying light meal.

* **Works best in a large (minimum 5 quart) slow cooker**

2 cups	cooked dried white kidney beans (see Basic Beans, page 231) or canned white kidney beans, drained and rinsed	500 mL
5 cups	lower-salt vegetable or chicken broth, divided	1.25 L
3 tbsp	olive oil, divided	45 mL
2	onions, finely chopped	2
2	carrots, peeled and diced	2
2	stalks celery, diced	2
4	cloves garlic, minced	4
¼ cup	finely chopped parsley	50 mL
1 tbsp	grated lemon zest	15 mL
1 tsp	finely chopped fresh rosemary leaves or dried rosemary leaves, crumbled	5 mL
¼ tsp	salt	1 mL
½ tsp	cracked black peppercorns	2 mL
2	potatoes, peeled and grated	2
4 cups	packed torn Swiss chard leaves (about 1 bunch) (see Tip, left)	1 L
1	long red chile pepper, minced, optional	1
3	thick slices day-old country-style bread	3
½ cup	freshly grated Parmesan cheese	125 mL

1. In a food processor, combine beans with 1 cup (250 mL) of the broth and purée until smooth. Set aside.

2. In a skillet, heat 1 tbsp (15 mL) of the oil over medium heat. Add onions, carrots and celery and cook, stirring, until carrots are softened, about 7 minutes. Add garlic, parsley, lemon zest, rosemary, salt and peppercorns and cook, stirring, for 1 minute. Add bean mixture and bring to a boil. Transfer mixture to stoneware.

NUTRIENTS PER SERVING	
Calories	228
Fat	7.5 g
Saturates	1.7 g
Polyunsaturates	0.7 g
Monounsaturates	4.5 g
Cholesterol	4 mg
Sodium	585 mg
Carbohydrate	31.6 g
Fiber	6.9 g
Protein	9.3 g

AMERICA'S EXCHANGES	
2	Starch
½	High-fat Meat

CANADA'S CHOICES	
1½	Carbohydrate
½	Meat and Alternatives
1	Fat

Make Ahead

Cook this soup overnight or the day before you intend to serve it. Refrigerate until you are ready to serve, then reheat in the oven. Ladle the soup into ovenproof bowls, drizzle with olive oil and sprinkle with Parmesan. Bake in a preheated oven (350°F/180°C) for about 30 minutes, until the top is lightly browned.

3. Stir in potatoes and remaining 4 cups (1 L) broth. Cover and cook on Low for 8 to 10 hours or on High for 4 to 5 hours, until vegetables are tender. Stir in Swiss chard, chile pepper, if using, and bread. Cover and cook on High for 30 minutes, until chard is cooked.

4. When ready to serve, ladle into bowls, breaking bread into pieces. Drizzle with remaining oil and sprinkle with Parmesan.

Mindful Morsels

In this traditional soup I've used Swiss chard, a relative of the beet family (the red stems of some chard varieties remind us of this relationship). Half a cup (125 mL) of cooked chard is an excellent source of beta carotene and also contains vitamin E, both of which also act as antioxidants. Together with other components of diets containing generous amounts of vegetables, antioxidants are believed to work to reduce the risk of some types of cancer.

MAKES 8 SERVINGS

Make Ahead

Harira can be partially prepared before it is cooked. Complete Step 1. Cover and refrigerate overnight or for up to 2 days. When you're ready to cook, continue with Step 2.

Harira

This traditional Moroccan soup, often made with lamb, is usually served during Ramadan at the end of a day of fasting. This vegetarian version is finished with a dollop of harissa, a spicy North African sauce, which adds flavor and punch. Served with whole grain bread, harira makes a great light meal.

• **Large (minimum 5 quart) slow cooker**

1 tbsp	olive oil	15 mL
2	onions, coarsely chopped	2
4	stalks celery, diced	4
2	cloves garlic, minced	2
1 tbsp	turmeric	15 mL
1 tbsp	grated lemon zest	15 mL
½ tsp	cracked black peppercorns	2 mL
1	can (28 oz/796 mL) diced tomatoes, including juice	1
4 cups	Basic Vegetable Stock or Homemade Chicken Stock (see recipes, pages 38 and 39) or lower-salt broth	1 L
1 cup	dried red lentils, rinsed	250 mL
1	can (14 oz/398 mL) chickpeas, drained and rinsed, or ½ cup (125 mL) dried chickpeas, soaked, cooked and drained (see Variation, page 231)	1
½ cup	finely chopped parsley	125 mL
	Harissa (see recipe, opposite)	

1. In a skillet, heat oil over medium heat for 30 seconds. Add onions and celery and cook, stirring, until celery is softened, about 5 minutes. Add garlic, turmeric, lemon zest and peppercorns and cook, stirring, for 1 minute. Add tomatoes with juice and bring to a boil. Transfer to slow cooker stoneware.

2. Add stock, lentils and chickpeas and stir well. Cover and cook on Low for 6 to 8 hours or on High for 3 to 4 hours, until mixture is hot and bubbly and lentils are tender. Stir in parsley. Ladle into bowls and pass the harissa at the table.

NUTRIENTS PER SERVING	
Calories	201
Fat	4.2 g
Saturates	0.6 g
Polyunsaturates	0.8 g
Monounsaturates	2.4 g
Cholesterol	0 mg
Sodium	314 mg
Carbohydrate	33.3 g
Fiber	7.0 g
Protein	10.2 g

AMERICA'S EXCHANGES	
1½	Starch
1	Vegetable
1	Lean Meat

CANADA'S CHOICES	
2	Carbohydrate
1	Meat and Alternatives

Tips

To prepare chiles for Harissa: Remove the stems and combine with 1 cup (250 mL) boiling water in a small bowl. Ensure they are submerged and set aside for 30 minutes, until soft. Drain and coarsely chop.

To toast seeds for Harissa: Combine caraway, coriander and cumin seeds in a dry skillet over medium heat. Cook, stirring, until fragrant, about 3 minutes. Immediately transfer to a mortar or a spice grinder and grind.

Harissa

In a mini-chopper, combine 3 reconstituted red chile peppers (see Tips, left), 2 tsp (10 mL) each toasted caraway and coriander seeds, 1 tsp (5 mL) toasted cumin seeds (see Tips, left), 2 reconstituted sun-dried tomatoes, 4 cloves garlic, $1\frac{1}{2}$ tbsp (22 mL) lemon juice, 1 tbsp (15 mL) sweet paprika and $\frac{1}{2}$ tsp (2 mL) salt and process until combined. Add 3 tbsp (45 mL) extra virgin olive oil and process until smooth and blended. Store, covered, in the refrigerator for up to 1 month, covering the paste with a bit of olive oil every time you use it. Makes $\frac{1}{3}$ cup (75 mL).

Mindful Morsels

A serving of this soup is an excellent source of the mineral potassium. Potassium works with sodium to help your body maintain a proper fluid balance, and although potassium is present in many foods, it is vulnerable to being depleted from the body. A diet high in refined foods is linked with potassium loss, as is the overconsumption of coffee. Prolonged diarrhea or the use of diuretics can also lead to potassium deficiencies, and boiling vegetables in large amounts of water causes the potassium to drain off.

Tips

Shred collard greens as if you were making a chiffonade of basil leaves. Remove the stems, including the thick vein that runs up the bottom of the leaf, and thoroughly wash the leaves by swishing them around in a sink full of warm water. On a cutting board, stack the leaves, 2 or 3 at a time. Roll them into a cigar shape and slice as thinly as you can.

Try a garnish of lean turkey kielbassa (or other lean cooked sausage). One tablespoon (15 mL), finely diced, counts as 1 Free Food/Extra.

Caldo Verde

This soup, which is Portuguese in origin, is usually made with white beans and kale. This version, which uses chickpeas and collard greens, is equally delicious and also lends itself to many adaptations. If you can't find collards, use kale, and feel free to substitute white beans for the chickpeas. Serve this as the centerpiece of a soup-and-salad meal. Add crusty whole grain bread or ciabatta and a salad of grated carrots with a lemon juice and extra virgin olive oil vinaigrette.

- **Large (minimum 5 quart) slow cooker**

1 tsp	cumin seeds	5 mL
1 tbsp	olive oil	15 mL
2	onions, finely chopped	2
2	carrots, peeled and diced	2
2	cloves garlic, minced	2
1/2 tsp	cracked black peppercorns	2 mL
6 cups	Homemade Chicken Stock (see recipe, page 39) or lower-salt chicken broth	1.5 L
2	cans (each 14 to 19 oz/398 to 540 mL) chickpeas, drained and rinsed, or 2 cups (500 mL) dried chickpeas, soaked, cooked and drained (see Variation, page 231)	2
2	potatoes, peeled and diced	2
2 tsp	paprika, dissolved in 2 tbsp (25 mL) lemon juice	10 mL
4 cups	shredded collard greens (about one 12 oz/375 g bunch) (see Tips, left)	1 L
	Red wine vinegar, optional	

1. In a large dry skillet over medium heat, toast cumin seeds, stirring, until fragrant and they just begin to brown, about 3 minutes. Immediately transfer to a mortar or a spice grinder and grind. Set aside.

2. In same skillet, heat oil over medium heat for 30 seconds. Add onions and carrots and cook, stirring, until carrots are softened, about 7 minutes. Add garlic, peppercorns and reserved cumin and cook, stirring, for 1 minute. Transfer to slow cooker stoneware. Add stock and chickpeas and stir well.

NUTRIENTS PER SERVING	
Calories	190
Fat	3.7 g
Saturates	0.6 g
Polyunsaturates	0.9 g
Monounsaturates	1.8 g
Cholesterol	5 mg
Sodium	243 mg
Carbohydrate	33.0 g
Fiber	6.1 g
Protein	7.9 g

AMERICA'S EXCHANGES	
2	Starch
1	Vegetable
1/2	Fat

CANADA'S CHOICES	
1 1/2	Carbohydrate
1/2	Meat and Alternatives

Make Ahead

This dish can be assembled before it is cooked. Complete Steps 1 and 2. Cover and refrigerate overnight or for up to 2 days. When you're ready to cook, continue with Step 3.

3. Add potatoes and stir well. Cover and cook on Low for 8 hours or on High for 4 hours, until potatoes are tender. If you prefer a smooth soup, working in batches, purée soup in a food processor or blender and return to slow cooker. (You can also do this in the stoneware using an immersion blender.) Stir in paprika mixture. Add collards, in batches, stirring each to submerge before adding the next batch. Cover and cook on High until collards are tender, about 30 minutes. Season to taste with vinegar, if using.

Mindful Morsels

One serving of this soup is an excellent source of vitamins A, B_6 and K and a good source of folacin, potassium and magnesium. Think of it as a steaming bowl of comfort. Many of the nutrients it contains, such as complex carbohydrates, vitamin B_6, folacin and magnesium, help your body manage stress.

Mushroom Lentil Soup

MAKES 8 SERVINGS

Tips

If you're using a strongly flavored dried mushroom, such as porcini, to make this soup, 2 tbsp (25 mL) will be sufficient. But if you're using a mixture of mushrooms, some of which may be more mildly flavored, you may need an additional 1 tbsp (15 mL) or so.

Lentils purchased in bulk may contain bits of dirt or discolored seeds. Before using, it is wise to rinse them thoroughly in a pot of water. Swish them around and remove any offending particles, then rinse thoroughly under cold running water.

If you prefer a creamier soup, after the soup has finished cooking, scoop out about 2 cups (500 mL) of the solids plus a little liquid and purée in a food processor. Return to the stoneware and continue as directed.

Make Ahead

This soup can be assembled before it is cooked. Complete Steps 1 and 2. Cover and refrigerate overnight or for up to 2 days. When you're ready to cook, continue with Step 3.

Lentils and mushrooms are a classic combination for a reason — they blend deliciously because each brings out the best features of the other. This hearty soup with its deep earthy flavors makes a great main course in a bowl. Serve it on those evenings when family members are coming and going at different times. Set out a loaf of whole grain bread and the fixin's for salad and let everyone help themselves.

- **Large (minimum 5 quart) slow cooker**

2 cups	hot water	500 mL
2 tbsp	dried wild mushrooms (see Tips, left)	25 mL
1 tbsp	olive oil	15 mL
1	onion, finely chopped	1
4	stalks celery, diced	4
2	carrots, peeled and diced	2
1 tsp	chili powder	5 mL
1	can (28 oz/796 mL) diced tomatoes, including juice	1
4 cups	Basic Vegetable Stock or Homemade Chicken Stock (see recipes, pages 38 and 39) or lower-salt broth	1 L
2 cups	brown or green lentils (see Tips, left)	500 mL
2 tbsp	freshly squeezed lemon juice	25 mL
	Freshly ground black pepper	
1 cup	low-fat plain yogurt, optional	250 mL
½ cup	finely chopped parsley leaves or chives	125 mL

1. In a heatproof bowl, combine hot water and dried mushrooms. Let stand for 30 minutes then strain through a fine sieve, reserving liquid. Pat mushrooms dry, chop finely and set aside.

2. In a large skillet, heat oil over medium heat for 30 seconds. Add onion, celery and carrots and cook, stirring, until carrots are softened, about 7 minutes. Add chili powder and reserved dried mushrooms and cook, stirring, for 1 minute. Add tomatoes, with juice, and reserved mushroom liquid and bring to a boil. Transfer to slow cooker stoneware.

3. Add stock and lentils. Cover and cook on Low for 8 to 10 hours or on High for 4 to 5 hours, until vegetables are tender. Stir in lemon and ground pepper. Ladle into bowls and drizzle each with 1 to 2 tbsp (15 to 25 mL) yogurt, if using. Garnish each serving with 1 tbsp (15 mL) parsley.

NUTRIENTS PER SERVING	
Calories	217
Fat	2.5 g
Saturates	0.4 g
Polyunsaturates	0.5 g
Monounsaturates	1.4 g
Cholesterol	0 mg
Sodium	188 mg
Carbohydrate	37.3 g
Fiber	7.9 g
Protein	14.2 g

AMERICA'S EXCHANGES	
1½	Starch
2	Vegetable
1	Very Lean Meat

CANADA'S CHOICES	
2	Carbohydrate
1	Meat and Alternatives

MAKES 8 SERVINGS

Tips

If you're using cayenne pepper, dissolve it in the lemon juice before adding to the slow cooker.

If you are using fresh spinach leaves in this recipe, take care to wash them thoroughly, as they can be quite gritty. To wash spinach: Fill a clean sink with lukewarm water. Remove the tough stems and submerge the tender leaves in the water, swishing to remove the grit. Rinse thoroughly in a colander under cold running water, checking carefully to ensure that no sand remains. If you are using frozen spinach in this recipe, thaw and squeeze the excess moisture out before adding to the slow cooker.

Make Ahead

This soup can be partially prepared before it is cooked. Complete Step 1. Cover and refrigerate for up to 2 days. When you're ready to cook, continue with the recipe.

Mediterranean Lentil Soup with Spinach

This delicious soup, delicately flavored with lemon and cumin, reminds me of hot, languid days under the Mediterranean sun. Serve it as a starter or add a green salad and warm country-style bread for a refreshing and nutritious light meal.

• **Works best in a large (minimum 5 quart) slow cooker**

1 tbsp	olive oil	15 mL
2	onions, chopped	2
2	stalks celery, chopped	2
2	large carrots, peeled and chopped	2
1	clove garlic, minced	1
1 tsp	cumin seeds, toasted and ground (see Tips, page 58)	5 mL
1 tsp	grated lemon zest	5 mL
6 cups	lower-salt vegetable or chicken broth	1.5 L
1	potato, peeled and grated	1
1 cup	green or brown lentils, rinsed	250 mL
2 tbsp	freshly squeezed lemon juice	25 mL
½ tsp	cayenne pepper, optional (see Tips, left)	2 mL
1 lb	fresh spinach, stems removed, or 1 package (10 oz/300 g) spinach leaves, thawed if frozen (see Tips, left)	500 g

1. In a skillet, heat oil over medium heat for 30 seconds. Add onions, celery and carrots and cook, stirring, until carrots are softened, about 7 minutes. Add garlic, toasted cumin and lemon zest and cook, stirring, for 1 minute. Transfer to slow cooker stoneware. Add broth.

2. Stir in potato and lentils. Cover and cook on Low for 8 to 10 hours or on High for 4 to 6 hours, until vegetables are tender. Add lemon juice and cayenne, if using, and stir. Add spinach. Cover and cook on High for 20 minutes, until spinach is cooked and mixture is hot and bubbly.

NUTRIENTS PER SERVING	
Calories	157
Fat	2.6 g
Saturates	0.3 g
Polyunsaturates	0.4 g
Monounsaturates	1.3 g
Cholesterol	0 mg
Sodium	396 mg
Carbohydrate	26.0 g
Fiber	6.0 g
Protein	9.2 g

AMERICA'S EXCHANGES	
1½	Starch
1	Vegetable
1	Lean Meat

CANADA'S CHOICES	
1	Carbohydrate
1	Meat and Alternatives

MAKES 8 SERVINGS

Tips

Traditional wisdom suggests that yellow split peas do not need to be soaked before cooking. However, I have found that without a good pre-soaking they are a bit tough.

Persillade counts as 1 Free Food/Extra.

Make Ahead

This soup can be partially prepared before it is cooked. Complete Steps 1 and 2. Cover and refrigerate overnight or for up to 2 days. When you're ready to cook, continue with Steps 3 and 4.

Variation

Instead of the persillade, top each serving of soup with a dollop of warm tomato sauce.

Greek-Style Split Pea Soup

This is a soup version of the Greek appetizer fava, a purée of yellow split peas often topped with capers or stewed tomatoes. Here I've suggested the addition of a persillade made with red wine vinegar as a flavor enhancer, but you can also finish the soup with a dollop of warm tomato sauce. For a smoother result, purée the soup after it has finished cooking.

- **Large (minimum 5 quart) slow cooker**

2 cups	yellow split peas (see Tips, left)	500 mL
1 tbsp	olive oil	15 mL
2	onions, finely chopped	2
4	stalks celery, diced	4
4	carrots, peeled and diced	4
4	cloves garlic, minced	4
1 tsp	dried oregano leaves, crumbled	5 mL
½ tsp	cracked black peppercorns	2 mL
6 cups	Enhanced Vegetable Stock (see Variation, page 38) or lower-salt vegetable broth	1.5 L

Persillade (optional)

1 cup	packed parsley leaves, finely chopped	250 mL
4	cloves garlic, minced	4
4 tsp	red wine vinegar	20 mL

1. In a large pot, combine split peas and 8 cups (2 L) cold water. Bring to a boil over medium-high heat and boil rapidly for 3 minutes. Turn off element and set aside for 1 hour. Drain and rinse thoroughly. Set aside.

2. In a skillet, heat oil over medium heat for 30 seconds. Add onions, celery and carrots and cook, stirring, until carrots are softened, about 7 minutes. Add garlic, oregano and peppercorns and cook, stirring, for 1 minute. Transfer to slow cooker stoneware. Add reserved split peas and stock and stir well.

3. Cover and cook on Low for 8 to 10 hours or on High for 4 to 5 hours, until peas are tender.

4. **Persillade (optional):** In a bowl, combine parsley, garlic and vinegar. (You can also make this in a mini-chopper.) Set aside at room temperature for 30 minutes to allow flavors to develop. To serve, ladle soup into individual bowls and garnish with persillade, if using.

NUTRIENTS PER SERVING	
Calories	230
Fat	2.4 g
Saturates	0.3 g
Polyunsaturates	0.5 g
Monounsaturates	1.4 g
Cholesterol	0 mg
Sodium	47 mg
Carbohydrate	39.5 g
Fiber	6.2 g
Protein	13.4 g

AMERICA'S EXCHANGES	
2	Starch
1	Vegetable
1	Very Lean Meat

CANADA'S CHOICES	
2	Carbohydrate
1	Meat and Alternatives

MAKES 8 SERVINGS

Make Ahead

Ideally, make this soup the day before you intend to serve it so it can chill overnight in the refrigerator.

Beet Soup with Lemongrass and Lime

This Thai-inspired soup, which is served cold, is elegant and refreshing. Its jewel-like appearance and intriguing flavors make it a perfect prelude to any meal. I especially like to serve it at summer dinners in the garden.

• **Works in slow cookers from 3½ to 6 quarts**

1 tbsp	olive oil	15 mL
1	onion, chopped	1
4	cloves garlic, minced	4
2 tbsp	minced gingerroot	25 mL
2	stalks lemongrass, trimmed, smashed and cut in half crosswise	2
2 tsp	cracked black peppercorns	10 mL
6	medium beets, peeled and chopped (about 2½ lbs/1.25 kg)	6
6 cups	Basic Vegetable Stock (see recipe, page 38) or lower-salt vegetable broth	1.5 L
1	red bell pepper, seeded and diced	1
1	long red chile pepper, seeded and diced, optional	1
	Zest and juice of 1 lime	
	Finely chopped cilantro	

1. In a skillet, heat oil over medium heat for 30 seconds. Add onion and cook, stirring, until softened, about 3 minutes. Add garlic, gingerroot, lemongrass and peppercorns and cook, stirring, for 1 minute. Transfer to slow cooker stoneware.

2. Add beets and stock. Cover and cook on Low for 8 hours or on High for 4 hours, until beets are tender. Add red pepper and chile pepper, if using. Cover and cook on High for 30 minutes, until peppers are tender. Remove lemongrass and discard.

3. Working in batches, purée soup in a food processor or blender. (You can also do this in the stoneware using an immersion blender.) Transfer to a large bowl. Stir in lime zest and juice. Chill thoroughly, preferably overnight.

4. When ready to serve, spoon into individual bowls and garnish with cilantro.

NUTRIENTS PER SERVING	
Calories	85
Fat	2.0 g
Saturates	0.3 g
Polyunsaturates	0.3 g
Monounsaturates	1.3 g
Cholesterol	0 mg
Sodium	85 mg
Carbohydrate	16.3 g
Fiber	2.9 g
Protein	2.4 g

AMERICA'S EXCHANGES	
1	Starch
½	Fat

CANADA'S CHOICES	
1	Carbohydrate
½	Fat

Cabbage Borscht

This hearty soup goes well with dark rye bread. I prefer the flavor when it's made with a combination of beef and lower-salt vegetable broth, but if you're a vegetarian, the lower-salt vegetable broth works well, too.

Tip

If you prefer a smoother soup, do not purée the vegetables in Step 2. Instead, wait until they have finished cooking, and purée the soup in the stoneware using an immersion blender before adding the vinegar and cabbage. Allow the soup time to reheat (cook on High for 10 or 15 minutes) before adding the cabbage to ensure that it cooks.

Make Ahead

This dish can be partially prepared before it is cooked. Complete Steps 1 and 2. Cover and refrigerate overnight or for up to 2 days. When you're ready to cook, continue with Step 3.

- **Large (minimum 6 quart) slow cooker**

1 tbsp	olive oil	15 mL
2	onions, finely chopped	2
4	stalks celery, diced	4
2	carrots, peeled and diced	2
4	cloves garlic, minced	4
1 tsp	caraway seeds	5 mL
1 tsp	salt	5 mL
½ tsp	cracked black peppercorns	2 mL
1	can (28 oz/796 mL) diced tomatoes, including juice	1
1 tbsp	brown sugar	15 mL
3	medium beets, peeled and diced	3
1	potato, peeled and diced	1
4 cups	Basic Vegetable Stock (see recipe, page 38) or 2 cups (500 mL) each lower-salt vegetable and beef broth	1 L
1 tbsp	red wine vinegar	15 mL
4 cups	finely shredded cabbage	1 L
	Light sour cream, optional	
	Finely chopped dill	

1. In a skillet, heat oil over medium heat for 30 seconds. Add onions, celery and carrots and cook, stirring, until carrots are softened, about 7 minutes. Add garlic, caraway seeds, salt and peppercorns and cook, stirring, for 1 minute.

2. Transfer to a food processor fitted with a metal blade (see Tip, left). Add half the tomatoes with juice and process until smooth. Transfer to slow cooker stoneware. Add remaining tomatoes, brown sugar, beets and potato to food processor and process until smooth. Transfer to slow cooker stoneware. Add stock.

3. Cover and cook on Low for 6 hours or on High for 3 hours, until vegetables are tender. Add vinegar and cabbage and stir well. Cover and cook on High for 20 to 30 minutes, until cabbage is tender. To serve, ladle into bowls, add 1 tbsp (15 mL) of sour cream to each, if using, and garnish with dill.

NUTRIENTS PER SERVING	
Calories	98
Fat	2.2 g
Saturates	0.3 g
Polyunsaturates	0.3 g
Monounsaturates	1.3 g
Cholesterol	0 mg
Sodium	487 mg
Carbohydrate	19.2 g
Fiber	3.3 g
Protein	2.8 g

AMERICA'S EXCHANGES	
1	Starch
1	Vegetable

CANADA'S CHOICES	
1	Carbohydrate
½	Fat

Gingery Carrot Soup with Orange and Parsley

In my book, carrots and ginger always make a superlative combination. Here, they are enhanced with zesty orange and a hit of earthy parsley to produce a delicious and versatile soup.

Tip

I provide a range of quantities for the ginger to suit individual tastes. If you find ginger a bit assertive, use the smaller amount. If you like its flavor, go for the larger quantity.

Make Ahead

This soup can be partially prepared before cooking. Complete Step 1, cover and refrigerate overnight or for up to 2 days. When you're ready to cook, continue with Steps 2 and 3.

- **Works in slow cookers from 3½ to 6 quarts**

1 tbsp	olive oil	15 mL
2	onions, chopped	2
2 to 3 tbsp	minced gingerroot (see Tip, left)	25 to 45 mL
1 tbsp	finely grated orange zest	15 mL
1 tsp	cracked black peppercorns	5 mL
2	bay leaves	2
6 cups	thinly sliced peeled carrots (about 6 large carrots)	1.5 L
4 cups	Basic Vegetable Stock or Homemade Chicken Stock (see recipes, pages 38 and 39) or lower-salt broth	1 L
1½ cups	freshly squeezed orange juice	375 mL
1 cup	packed parsley leaves	250 mL

1. In a skillet, heat oil over medium heat for 30 seconds. Add onions and cook, stirring, until softened, about 3 minutes. Add gingerroot, orange zest, peppercorns and bay leaves and cook, stirring, for 1 minute. Transfer to slow cooker stoneware. Add carrots and stock and stir well.

2. Cover and cook on Low for 8 hours or on High for 4 hours, until carrots are tender. Add orange juice and parsley. Cover and cook on High for 20 minutes, until heated through. Discard bay leaves.

3. Working in batches, purée soup in a food processor or blender. (You can also do this in the stoneware using an immersion blender.) Ladle into serving bowls and serve hot.

NUTRIENTS PER SERVING	
Calories	88
Fat	2.1 g
Saturates	0.3 g
Polyunsaturates	0.3 g
Monounsaturates	1.3 g
Cholesterol	0 mg
Sodium	58 mg
Carbohydrate	16.8 g
Fiber	3.0 g
Protein	1.8 g

AMERICA'S EXCHANGES	
½	Fruit
2	Vegetable
½	Fat

CANADA'S CHOICES	
1	Carbohydrate
½	Fat

Soup à la Crécy

MAKES 8 SERVINGS

Tips

To clean leeks: Fill a sink full of lukewarm water. Split the leeks in half lengthwise and submerge them in the water, swishing them around to remove all traces of dirt. Transfer to a colander and rinse thoroughly under cold water.

Store brown rice in the refrigerator or use it within a month of purchase. The bran layer contains oil, which, although healthy, becomes rancid when kept at room temperature for a long period.

Make Ahead

This dish can be partially prepared before it is cooked. Complete Step 1. Cover and refrigerate for up to 2 days. When you're ready to cook, continue with the recipe.

In French cooking, "crécy" is a term for certain dishes containing carrots. In my book, this soup, which may be thickened with potatoes or rice, is one of the tastiest. This classic soup makes a nice centerpiece for a light soup-and-salad dinner accompanied with dark rye bread. It also makes an elegant first course for a more sophisticated meal.

* **Works best in a large (minimum 5 quart) slow cooker**

1 tbsp	olive oil	15 mL
2	leeks, white part with just a bit of green, cleaned and thinly sliced (see Tips, left)	2
4 cups	thinly sliced peeled carrots (about 1 lb/500 g)	1 L
2 tsp	dried thyme leaves, crumbled	10 mL
1 tsp	cracked black peppercorns	5 mL
2	bay leaves	2
6 cups	lower-salt vegetable or chicken broth	1.5 L
½ cup	brown rice (see Tips, left)	125 mL
½ cup	finely chopped parsley or snipped chives	125 mL

1. In a large skillet, heat oil over medium heat for 30 seconds. Add leeks and carrots and cook, stirring, until carrots are softened, about 7 minutes. Add thyme, peppercorns and bay leaves and cook, stirring, for 1 minute. Transfer to slow cooker stoneware. Add broth and stir well.

2. Stir in rice. Cover and cook on Low for 8 hours or on High for 4 hours, until carrots are tender. Discard bay leaves.

3. Working in batches, purée soup in a food processor or blender. (You can also do this in the stoneware using an immersion blender.) Ladle into individual serving bowls, garnish with parsley and serve hot.

NUTRIENTS PER SERVING	
Calories	123
Fat	2.7 g
Saturates	0.3 g
Polyunsaturates	0.4 g
Monounsaturates	1.4 g
Cholesterol	0 mg
Sodium	393 mg
Carbohydrate	22.7 g
Fiber	4.2 g
Protein	2.9 g

AMERICA'S EXCHANGES	
2	Vegetable
1	Starch

CANADA'S CHOICES	
1	Carbohydrate
½	Fat

Chestnut Soup

French in origin, this soup makes an elegant starter to any meal. In France, chestnut soup is often accentuated with a licorice-flavored herb such as chervil or tarragon. Here, I have added the Chinese spice star anise.

MAKES 6 SERVINGS

Tip

If you are using prepared chestnut purée in this recipe, check the label to make sure it doesn't contain sugar. Some versions of this product are destined for dessert rather than main course use. Canned purée is very congealed and you'll need to soften it up a bit before adding to the broth. I suggest breaking it into little pieces and beating it in a bowl with a bit of the hot broth, or puréeing it in a food processor.

Make Ahead

This dish can be partially prepared before it is cooked. Complete Steps 1 and 2. Cover and refrigerate overnight or for up to 2 days. When you're ready to cook, continue with Step 3.

- **Works in slow cookers from 3½ to 6 quarts**

Garlic Croutons

1 tbsp	olive oil	15 mL
2	cloves garlic, minced	2
1	slice country-style bread, cut into ¼-inch (0.5 cm) cubes	1
1 tbsp	olive oil	15 mL
⅓ cup	minced onion	75 mL
2	carrots, peeled and diced	2
2	stalks celery, diced	2
1	whole star anise	1
¼ tsp	freshly ground black pepper	1 mL
4 cups	Basic Vegetable Stock or Homemade Chicken Stock (see recipes, pages 38 and 39) or lower-salt broth	1 L
1 cup	unsweetened chestnut purée (see Tip, left)	250 mL
1 tbsp	chopped fresh tarragon, chervil or parsley	15 mL
1 tbsp	port wine, optional	15 mL

1. **Garlic Croutons:** In a skillet, heat oil over medium heat for 30 seconds. Add garlic and cook, stirring, for 1 minute. Add bread and cook, stirring, until golden, about 2 minutes. Drain on paper towel–lined plate. If not using immediately, transfer to an airtight container. Set aside until ready to use.

2. In a skillet, heat oil over medium heat for 30 seconds. Add onion, carrots and celery and cook, stirring, until softened, about 7 minutes. Add star anise and black pepper and cook, stirring, for 1 minute. Transfer to slow cooker stoneware. Stir in stock.

3. Cover and cook on Low for 6 to 8 hours or on High for 3 to 4 hours, until vegetables are very tender. Stir in chestnut purée and tarragon. Cover and cook for 30 minutes, until flavors meld. Working in batches, purée soup in a food processor or blender. (You can also do this in the stoneware using an immersion blender.) Stir in port wine, if using. Ladle into bowls. Garnish with croutons.

NUTRIENTS PER SERVING	
Calories	156
Fat	6.2 g
Saturates	1.0 g
Polyunsaturates	0.9 g
Monounsaturates	3.9 g
Cholesterol	13 mg
Sodium	83 mg
Carbohydrate	21.8 g
Fiber	4.8 g
Protein	4.0 g

AMERICA'S EXCHANGES	
1	Starch
1	Vegetable
1	Fat

CANADA'S CHOICES	
1	Carbohydrate
1	Fat

Southwestern Corn and Roasted Red Pepper Soup

MAKES 8 SERVINGS

Although the roots of this soup lie deep in the heart of Tex-Mex cuisine, it is elegant enough for even the most gracious occasion. Hot sourdough bread makes a perfect accompaniment.

Tips

To toast cumin seeds: Place seeds in a dry skillet over medium heat, stirring, until fragrant, about 3 minutes. Immediately transfer to a mortar or a spice grinder and grind. If you prefer to use ground cumin, substitute half of the quantity called for.

To roast peppers: Preheat oven to 400°F (200°C). Place pepper(s) on a baking sheet and roast, turning two or three times, until the skin on all sides is blackened. (This will take about 25 minutes.) Transfer pepper(s) to a heatproof bowl. Cover with a plate and let stand until cool. Remove and, using a sharp knife, lift off skins. Discard skins, stem and core and slice according to recipe instructions.

- **Works best in a large (minimum 5 quart) slow cooker**

1 tbsp	olive oil	15 mL
1	large onion, finely chopped	1
6	cloves garlic, minced	6
1 tbsp	cumin seeds, toasted and ground (see Tips, left)	15 mL
1 tbsp	chopped fresh rosemary leaves or dried rosemary, crumbled	15 mL
1	bay leaf	1
½ tsp	salt	2 mL
½ tsp	cracked black peppercorns	2 mL
6 cups	lower-salt vegetable or chicken broth	1.5 L
1	dried New Mexico, ancho or guajillo chile pepper	1
1 cup	boiling water	250 mL
1	jalapeño pepper, seeded and coarsely chopped, optional	1
4 cups	corn kernels, thawed if frozen	1 L
2	red bell peppers, roasted and cut into ½-inch (1 cm) cubes (see Tips, left)	2
½ cup	whipping (35%) cream	125 mL
	Finely chopped parsley or cilantro	

1. In a skillet, heat oil over medium heat for 30 seconds. Add onion and cook, stirring, until softened, about 3 minutes. Add garlic, toasted cumin, rosemary, bay leaf, salt and peppercorns and cook, stirring, for 1 minute. Transfer to slow cooker stoneware. Add broth and stir well.

2. Cover and cook on Low for 6 to 8 hours or on High for 3 to 4 hours, until flavors meld.

NUTRIENTS PER SERVING	
Calories	180
Fat	8.1 g
Saturates	3.6 g
Polyunsaturates	0.7 g
Monounsaturates	2.9 g
Cholesterol	19 mg
Sodium	505 mg
Carbohydrate	26.1 g
Fiber	3.7 g
Protein	4.4 g

AMERICA'S EXCHANGES	
1½	Starch
1	Vegetable
1½	Fat

CANADA'S CHOICES	
1½	Carbohydrate
1½	Fat

This soup can be partially prepared before it is cooked. Complete Step 1. Cover and refrigerate for up to 2 days. When you're ready to cook, continue with the recipe.

3. Half an hour before soup has finished cooking, in a heatproof bowl, soak dried chile pepper in boiling water for 30 minutes, weighing down with a cup to ensure it remains submerged. Drain, discarding soaking liquid and stem, and chop coarsely. Transfer to a blender. Add 1 cup (250 mL) of broth from the soup and the jalapeño pepper, if using, and purée. Add to slow cooker and stir well. Add corn, roasted red pepper and whipping cream. Cover and cook on High for 30 minutes, until corn is tender. Discard bay leaf. Spoon into individual bowls and garnish with parsley.

Mindful Morsels

The rich color of red bell peppers (also known as sweet red peppers) lets us know that this tasty, versatile vegetable is high in important nutrients. A medium red pepper contains only about 30 calories and is an excellent source of both vitamin A (mostly as beta carotene) and vitamin C. In fact, ounce for ounce, red peppers contain more vitamin C than oranges. Both beta carotene and vitamin C act as antioxidants; consumed as part of a healthy diet, they may help to prevent some age-related ailments.

Leafy Greens Soup

This delicious country-style soup is French in origin and based on the classic combination of leeks and potatoes, with the addition of healthful leafy greens. Sorrel, which has an intriguing but bitter taste, adds depth to the flavor. Sorrel is available from specialty greengrocers or at farmers' markets during the summer, but if you're unsuccessful in locating it, arugula or parsley also work well in this recipe.

Tip

To clean leeks: Fill a sink full of lukewarm water. Split the leeks in half lengthwise and submerge them in the water, swishing them around to remove all traces of dirt. Transfer to a colander and rinse thoroughly under cold water.

Make Ahead

This soup can be partially prepared before it is cooked. Complete Step 1, cover and refrigerate overnight or for up to 2 days. When you're ready to cook, continue with Steps 2 and 3.

- Large (minimum 5 quart) slow cooker

1 tbsp	butter or olive oil	15 mL
1 tbsp	olive oil	15 mL
6	small leeks, white and light green parts only, cleaned and thinly sliced (see Tip, left)	6
4	cloves garlic, minced	4
1 tsp	salt	5 mL
1 tsp	dried tarragon	5 mL
½ tsp	cracked black peppercorns	2 mL
6 cups	Basic Vegetable Stock or Homemade Chicken Stock (see recipes, pages 38 and 39) or lower-salt broth	1.5 L
3	medium potatoes, peeled and cut into ½-inch (1 cm) cubes	3
4 cups	packed torn Swiss chard leaves (about 1 bunch)	1 L
1 cup	packed torn sorrel, arugula or parsley leaves	250 mL
	Half-and-half (10%) cream, optional	

1. In a large skillet over medium heat, melt butter and olive oil. Add leeks and cook, stirring, until softened, about 5 minutes. Add garlic, salt, tarragon and peppercorns and cook, stirring, for 1 minute. Add stock and bring to a boil. Transfer to slow cooker stoneware.

2. Stir in potatoes. Cover and cook on Low for 8 hours or on High for 4 hours, until potatoes are tender. Add Swiss chard and sorrel, in batches, stirring after each to submerge the leaves in the liquid. Cover and cook on High for 20 minutes, until greens are tender.

3. Working in batches, purée soup in a food processor or blender. (You can also do this in the stoneware using an immersion blender.) Spoon into individual serving bowls and drizzle each with 1 tbsp (15 mL) cream, if using.

NUTRIENTS PER SERVING	
Calories	122
Fat	3.5 g
Saturates	1.2 g
Polyunsaturates	0.4 g
Monounsaturates	1.7 g
Cholesterol	5 mg
Sodium	475 mg
Carbohydrate	21.8 g
Fiber	5.1 g
Protein	3.6 g

AMERICA'S EXCHANGES	
1	Starch
1	Vegetable
½	Fat

CANADA'S CHOICES	
1	Carbohydrate
½	Fat

MAKES 6 SERVINGS

Tips

If you are making this soup for vegetarians, omit the bacon and heat the 1 tbsp (15 mL) olive oil in a skillet over medium heat for 30 seconds. Add the onions and continue with the recipe.

You can use any kind of paprika in this recipe: regular, hot, which produces a nicely peppery version, or smoked, which adds a delicious note of smokiness to the soup. If you have regular paprika and would like a bit a heat, dissolve ¼ tsp (1 mL) cayenne pepper in the lemon juice along with the paprika.

Make ahead

This soup can be partially prepared before it is cooked. Complete Steps 1 and 2. Cover and refrigerate for up to 2 days. When you're ready to cook, continue with the recipe.

NUTRIENTS PER SERVING	
Calories	155
Fat	5.2 g
Saturates	1.1 g
Polyunsaturates	0.7 g
Monounsaturates	2.7 g
Cholesterol	4 mg
Sodium	404 mg
Carbohydrate	23.8 g
Fiber	3.4 g
Protein	5.1 g

Creamy Onion Soup with Kale

There is no cream in this delicious soup — unless you decide to drizzle a bit over individual servings. The creaminess is achieved with the addition of potatoes, which are puréed into the soup, providing it with a velvety texture.

• **Works best in a large (minimum 5 quart) slow cooker**

4	slices bacon (see Tips, left)	4
1 tbsp	olive oil	15 mL
4	onions, thinly sliced	4
2	cloves garlic, minced	2
1 tsp	grated lemon zest	5 mL
½ tsp	cracked black peppercorns	2 mL
1	bay leaf	1
4	whole allspice	4
4 cups	lower-salt vegetable or chicken broth	1 L
3	medium potatoes, peeled and diced	3
1 tsp	paprika, dissolved in 2 tbsp (25 mL) lemon juice (see Tips, left)	5 mL
4 cups	chopped kale	1 L

1. In a skillet, cook bacon over medium-high heat until crisp. Drain on paper towel and crumble. Cover and refrigerate until ready to use. Drain fat from pan.

2. Reduce heat to medium, add olive oil and heat for 30 seconds. Add onions to pan and cook, stirring, until softened, about 5 minutes. Add garlic, lemon zest, peppercorns, bay leaf and allspice and cook, stirring, for 1 minute. Transfer to slow cooker stoneware. Add broth and stir well.

3. Stir in potatoes. Cover and cook on Low for 8 hours or on High for 4 hours, until potatoes are tender. Discard bay leaf and allspice. Stir in paprika solution, kale and reserved bacon. Cover and cook on High for 20 minutes, until kale is tender. Working in batches, purée soup in a food processor or blender. (You can also do this in the stoneware using an immersion blender.) Serve immediately.

AMERICA'S EXCHANGES	
2	Vegetable
1	Starch
1	Fat

CANADA'S CHOICES	
1½	Carbohydrate
1	Fat

MAKES 8 SERVINGS

Tips

To clean leeks: Fill a sink full of lukewarm water. Split the leeks in half lengthwise and submerge them in the water, swishing them around to remove all traces of dirt. Transfer to a colander and rinse thoroughly under cold water.

If you prefer, use 1 red and 1 green bell pepper.

New World Leek and Sweet Potato Soup

I call this soup "new world" because it's a variation on the classic French leek and potato soup, using sweet potatoes and peppers, two ingredients that Christopher Columbus introduced to Europe during his explorations of the Americas.

- **Large (minimum 5 quart) slow cooker**

1 tbsp	cumin seeds	15 mL
1 tbsp	olive oil	15 mL
4	large leeks, white part with just a bit of green, cleaned and thinly sliced (see Tips, left)	4
4	cloves garlic, minced	4
½ tsp	cracked black peppercorns	2 mL
6 cups	Basic Vegetable Stock or Homemade Chicken Stock (see recipes, pages 38 and 39) or lower-salt broth	1.5 L
2 lbs	sweet potatoes, peeled and cut into 1-inch (2.5 cm) cubes (about 3 potatoes)	1 kg
2	green bell peppers, diced (see Tips, left)	2
1	long red chile pepper, minced, optional	1
½ cup	whipping (35%) cream or soy milk	125 mL
	Roasted red pepper strips, optional	
	Finely snipped chives	

1. In a large dry skillet over medium heat, toast cumin seeds, stirring, until fragrant and they just begin to brown, about 3 minutes. Immediately transfer to a mortar or a spice grinder and grind. Set aside.

2. In same skillet, heat oil over medium heat for 30 seconds. Add leeks and cook, stirring, until softened, about 5 minutes. Add garlic, peppercorns and reserved cumin and cook, stirring, for 1 minute. Transfer to slow cooker stoneware. Add stock.

3. Add sweet potatoes. Cover and cook on Low for 7 to 8 hours or on High for 3 to 4 hours, until potatoes are tender. Add green peppers and chile pepper, if using. Cover and cook on High for 20 to 30 minutes, until peppers are tender.

NUTRIENTS PER SERVING	
Calories	222
Fat	8.4 g
Saturates	3.8 g
Polyunsaturates	0.8 g
Monounsaturates	3.2 g
Cholesterol	34 mg
Sodium	44 mg
Carbohydrate	33.5 g
Fiber	4.2 g
Protein	5.1 g

AMERICA'S EXCHANGES	
1½	Starch
2	Vegetable
1½	Fat

CANADA'S CHOICES	
2	Carbohydrate
1½	Fat

Make Ahead

This dish can be partially prepared before it is cooked. Complete Steps 1 and 2. Cover and refrigerate overnight or for up to 2 days. When you're ready to cook, continue with Steps 3 and 4.

4. Working in batches, purée soup in a food processor or blender. (You can also do this in the stoneware using an immersion blender.) To serve, ladle soup into bowls, drizzle with cream and garnish each with 2 thin roasted red pepper strips, if using, and chives.

Mindful Morsels

One serving of this soup is an excellent source of vitamin A, much of which comes from the sweet potatoes. Sweet potatoes are one of the best sources of beta carotene, which our bodies convert to vitamin A. The more colorful a fruit or vegetable is, the higher it is in vitamins. Remember that most vegetables are also low in calories and carbohydrate — $\frac{1}{2}$ cup (125 mL) of a cooked vegetable (or 1 cup/250 mL of salad greens) usually counts as a Free Food/Extra. Aim for at least seven servings per day, and be sure to include at least one serving of an orange vegetable (such as the sweet potatoes in this recipe) and a dark green one such as broccoli, romaine lettuce or spinach.

Mushroom Soup with Millet

Enhancing this soup with dried mushrooms and their soaking liquid produces a deeply flavored broth that lingers on the taste buds. A splash of soy sauce moves the flavor profile to the east. If you prefer a creamy finish, add a drizzle of low-fat plain yogurt.

Tips

Two tablespoons (25 mL) of dried mushrooms are about half of a ½ oz (14 g) package.

Millet is available in natural food stores. Like lentils, some millet may contain bits of dirt or discolored grains. If your millet looks grimy, rinse it thoroughly in a pot of water before using. Swish it around and remove any offending particles, then rinse under cold running water. If you can't find millet, you can also make this soup with brown rice or a mixture of wild and brown rice (see Variation, below) and still benefit from including whole grains in your diet.

If you prefer, make this soup using 5 cups (1.25 L) lower-salt beef broth and 1 cup (250 mL) white wine or water, instead of the vegetable stock.

Variation

Mushroom Soup with Rice: Substitute the millet with ³⁄₄ cup (175 mL) rinsed brown rice or a mixture of wild and brown rice.

- **Large (minimum 5 quart) slow cooker**

3 cups	hot water	750 mL
2 tbsp	dried wild mushrooms (see Tips, left)	25 mL
½ cup	millet (see Tips, left)	125 mL
1 tbsp	olive oil	15 mL
2	onions, finely chopped	2
6	cloves garlic, minced	6
1 tbsp	minced gingerroot	15 mL
½ tsp	cracked black peppercorns	2 mL
2 lbs	button mushrooms, trimmed and thinly sliced	1 kg
6 cups	Basic Vegetable Stock (see recipe, page 38) or 3 cups (750 mL) each lower-salt vegetable broth and water	1.5 L
2	bay leaves	2
¼ cup	light (reduced-sodium) soy or tamari sauce	50 mL
	Low-fat plain yogurt, optional	
½ cup	finely chopped green onions or parsley leaves	125 mL

1. In a heatproof bowl, combine hot water and dried mushrooms. Let stand for 30 minutes, then strain through a fine sieve, reserving liquid. Pat mushrooms dry, chop finely and set aside.

2. In a large skillet over medium heat, toast millet, stirring, until fragrant and beginning to turn golden, about 3 minutes. Transfer to slow cooker stoneware.

3. In same skillet, heat oil over medium heat for 30 seconds. Add onions and cook, stirring, until softened, about 3 minutes. Add reserved mushrooms, garlic, gingerroot and peppercorns and cook, stirring, for 1 minute. Add reserved mushroom liquid and bring to a boil. Transfer to slow cooker stoneware.

NUTRIENTS PER SERVING	
Calories	108
Fat	2.6 g
Saturates	0.4 g
Polyunsaturates	0.5 g
Monounsaturates	1.3 g
Cholesterol	0 mg
Sodium	307 mg
Carbohydrate	18.8 g
Fiber	3.7 g
Protein	4.2 g

AMERICA'S EXCHANGES	
½	Starch
2	Vegetable
½	Fat

CANADA'S CHOICES	
1	Carbohydrate
½	Fat

Make Ahead

This soup can be assembled before it is cooked. Complete Steps 1 through 3. Cover and refrigerate for up to 2 days. When you're ready to cook, continue with Step 4.

4. Add button mushrooms, stock, bay leaves and soy sauce. Cover and cook on Low for 6 to 8 hours or on High for 3 to 4 hours, until millet is tender. Discard bay leaves. Ladle into individual bowls, drizzle with yogurt, if using, and garnish each serving with 1 tbsp (15 mL) green onion.

Mindful Morsels

I've included millet in this recipe because it's a nutritious whole grain that most people don't often eat. One-half cup (125 mL) of cooked millet contains almost 3 g of fiber and less than 1 g of fat; it's a good source of magnesium and also supplies thiamine, niacin, vitamin B_6, folacin, manganese, phosphorus and zinc. The slowly released low-glycemic-index carbohydrate in whole grains causes a smaller increase in blood glucose than many other carbohydrate-containing foods. Whole grains are also more filling than their refined versions. As an added bonus, a diet high in whole grains is associated with a decreased risk of heart disease, among other benefits.

Vichyssoise with Celery Root and Watercress

MAKES 10 SERVINGS

Tips

To clean leeks: Fill a sink full of lukewarm water. Split the leeks in half lengthwise and submerge them in the water, swishing them around to remove all traces of dirt. Transfer to a colander and rinse thoroughly under cold water.

Since celery root oxidizes quickly on contact with air, be sure to use as soon as you have peeled and chopped it, or toss with 1 tbsp (15 mL) lemon juice to prevent discoloration.

To cool the soup more quickly, transfer it to a large bowl before refrigerating.

Make Ahead

This dish can be partially prepared before it is cooked. Complete Step 1. Cover and refrigerate overnight or for up to 2 days. When you're ready to cook, continue with Steps 2 and 3.

This refreshing soup is delicious, easy to make and can be a prelude to the most sophisticated meal. More nutritious than traditional vichyssoise, it has a pleasing nutty flavor. In the summer, I aim to have leftovers in the refrigerator and treat myself with a yummy afternoon snack.

* **Large (minimum 5 quart) slow cooker**

1 tbsp	olive oil	15 mL
3	leeks, white and light green parts only, cleaned and coarsely chopped (see Tips, left)	3
2	cloves garlic, minced	2
½ tsp	cracked black peppercorns	2 mL
6 cups	Basic Vegetable Stock or Homemade Chicken Stock (see recipes, pages 38 and 39) or lower-salt broth	1.5 L
1	large celery root, peeled and sliced (see Tips, left)	1
2	bunches (each about 4 oz/125 g) watercress, tough parts of the stems removed	2
½ cup	whipping (35%) cream	125 mL
	Watercress sprigs, optional	

1. In a skillet, heat oil over medium heat for 30 seconds. Add leeks and cook, stirring, until softened, about 5 minutes. Add garlic and peppercorns and cook, stirring, for 1 minute. Transfer to slow cooker stoneware. Add stock and stir well.

2. Stir in celery root. Cover and cook on Low for 6 hours or on High for 3 hours, until celery root is tender. Stir in watercress until wilted.

3. Working in batches, purée mixture in a food processor or blender. (You can also do this in the stoneware using an immersion blender.) Stir in cream and refrigerate until thoroughly chilled, about 4 hours (see Tips, left). To serve, ladle into bowls and garnish with watercress sprigs, if using.

NUTRIENTS PER SERVING	
Calories	103
Fat	6.4 g
Saturates	3.0 g
Polyunsaturates	0.4 g
Monounsaturates	2.5 g
Cholesterol	27 mg
Sodium	85 mg
Carbohydrate	9.2 g
Fiber	2.4 g
Protein	3.6 g

AMERICA'S EXCHANGES	
2	Vegetable
1	Fat

CANADA'S CHOICES	
½	Carbohydrate
1	Fat

MAKES 8 SERVINGS

Tip

If you are using large parsnips in this recipe, cut away the woody core and discard.

Make Ahead

This dish can be partially prepared before it is cooked. Complete Steps 1 and 2. Cover and refrigerate overnight or for up to 2 days. When you're ready to cook, continue with Steps 3 and 4.

Curried Parsnip Soup with Green Peas

Flavorful and elegant, this soup makes a great introduction to a meal.

- **Large (minimum 5 quart) slow cooker**

2 tsp	cumin seeds	10 mL
1 tsp	coriander seeds	5 mL
1 tbsp	olive oil or extra virgin coconut oil	15 mL
2	onions, finely chopped	2
4	cloves garlic, minced	4
½ tsp	cracked black peppercorns	2 mL
1	piece (1 inch/2.5 cm) cinnamon stick	1
1	bay leaf	1
6 cups	Basic Vegetable Stock or Homemade Chicken Stock (see recipes, pages 38 and 39) or lower-salt broth	1.5 L
4 cups	sliced peeled parsnips (about 1 lb/500 g) (see Tip, left)	1 L
2 tsp	curry powder, dissolved in 4 tsp (20 mL) freshly squeezed lemon juice	10 mL
2 cups	sweet green peas, thawed if frozen	500 mL
⅓ cup	whipping (35%) cream	75 mL

1. In a large dry skillet over medium heat, toast cumin and coriander seeds, stirring, until fragrant and cumin seeds just begin to brown, about 3 minutes. Immediately transfer to a mortar or a spice grinder and grind. Set aside.

2. In same skillet, heat oil over medium heat for 30 seconds. Add onions and cook, stirring, until softened, about 3 minutes. Add garlic, peppercorns, cinnamon stick, bay leaf and reserved cumin and coriander and cook, stirring, for 1 minute. Transfer to slow cooker stoneware. Add stock and parsnips and stir well.

3. Cover and cook on Low for 6 hours or on High for 3 hours, until parsnips are tender. Discard cinnamon stick and bay leaf.

4. Working in batches, purée soup in a food processor or blender. (You can also do this in the stoneware using an immersion blender.) Return to slow cooker stoneware. Add curry powder solution, green peas and whipping cream. Cover and cook on High for 20 minutes, until peas are tender and cream is heated through.

NUTRIENTS PER SERVING	
Calories	146
Fat	5.7 g
Saturates	2.5 g
Polyunsaturates	0.4 g
Monounsaturates	2.5 g
Cholesterol	13 mg
Sodium	40 mg
Carbohydrate	22.2 g
Fiber	4.3 g
Protein	3.4 g

AMERICA'S EXCHANGES	
1	Starch
1	Vegetable
1	Fat

CANADA'S CHOICES	
1	Carbohydrate
1	Fat

Thai-Style Pumpkin Soup

This soup is both versatile and delicious. It has an exotic combination of flavors and works well as a prelude to a meal. If you prefer a more substantial soup, top each serving with cooked shrimp or scallops.

Tips

Most vegetable oils contain only a small amount of saturated fat and varying amounts of poly- and monounsaturated fatty acids. Coconut oil is one of the few exceptions. Because of its high saturated fat level, it should be used sparingly, and only when its distinctive flavor is important to the dish. (See also page 153.)

Coconut cream is the thick part of the liquid that accumulates on the top of canned coconut milk. Scoop out the required quantity, then stir the remainder well for use in the soup.

Make Ahead

This soup can be partially prepared before it is cooked. Complete Step 1. Cover and refrigerate overnight or for up to 2 days. When you're ready to cook, continue with Steps 2 and 3.

- **Large (minimum 6 quart) slow cooker**

1 tbsp	olive oil or extra virgin coconut oil	15 mL
2	onions, finely chopped	2
4	cloves garlic, minced	4
2 tbsp	minced gingerroot	25 mL
1 tsp	cracked black peppercorns	5 mL
2	stalks lemongrass, trimmed, smashed and cut in half crosswise	2
1 tbsp	cumin seeds, toasted and ground (see Tips, page 73)	15 mL
8 cups	cubed peeled pumpkin or other orange squash (2-inch/5 cm cubes)	2 L
6 cups	Basic Vegetable Stock or Homemade Chicken Stock (see recipes, pages 38 and 39) or prepared lower-salt broth	1.5 L
1 cup	coconut milk	250 mL
1 tsp	Thai red curry paste	5 mL
	Finely grated zest and juice of 1 lime	
¼ cup	toasted pumpkin seeds, optional	50 mL
	Cherry tomatoes, halved, optional	
	Finely chopped cilantro	

1. In a skillet, heat oil over medium heat for 30 seconds. Add onions and cook, stirring, until softened, about 3 minutes. Add garlic, gingerroot, peppercorns, lemongrass and toasted cumin and cook, stirring, for 1 minute. Transfer to slow cooker stoneware. Add pumpkin and stock.

2. Cover and cook on Low for 8 hours or on High for 4 hours, until pumpkin is tender. Skim off 1 tbsp (15 mL) of the coconut cream (see Tips, left). In a small bowl, combine with curry paste and blend well. Add to slow cooker along with remaining coconut milk and lime zest and juice. Cover and cook on High until heated through, about 20 minutes. Discard lemongrass.

3. Working in batches, purée soup in a food processor or blender. (You can also do this in the stoneware using an immersion blender.) Ladle into bowls and garnish with pumpkin seeds and/or tomatoes, if using, and cilantro.

NUTRIENTS PER SERVING	
Calories	130
Fat	8.4 g
Saturates	5.7 g
Polyunsaturates	0.4 g
Monounsaturates	1.8 g
Cholesterol	0 mg
Sodium	9 mg
Carbohydrate	14.3 g
Fiber	2.4 g
Protein	2.5 g

AMERICA'S EXCHANGES	
½	Starch
1	Vegetable
1½	Fat

CANADA'S CHOICES	
1	Carbohydrate
1½	Fat

MAKES 8 SERVINGS

Make Ahead

This soup can be partially prepared the night before it is cooked. Complete Step 1. Cover and refrigerate for up to 2 days. When you're ready to cook, continue with the recipe.

Butternut Apple Soup with Swiss Cheese

Topped with melted cheese, this creamy and delicious soup is an ideal antidote to a blustery day.

• **Works best in a large (minimum 5 quart) slow cooker**

1 tbsp	olive oil	15 mL
2	onions, chopped	2
4	cloves garlic, minced	4
2 tsp	dried rosemary leaves, crumbled, or 1 tbsp (15 mL) chopped fresh rosemary leaves	10 mL
½ tsp	cracked black peppercorns	2 mL
5 cups	lower-salt vegetable or chicken broth	1.25 L
1	butternut squash, peeled, seeded and cut into 1-inch (2.5 cm) cubes (about 2½ lbs/1.25 kg)	1
2	tart apples, such as Granny Smith, cored, peeled and coarsely chopped	2
1 cup	shredded light Swiss cheese	250 mL
½ cup	finely chopped walnuts, optional	125 mL

1. In a skillet, heat oil over medium heat for 30 seconds. Add onions and cook, stirring, until softened, about 3 minutes. Add garlic, rosemary and peppercorns and cook, stirring, for 1 minute. Transfer to slow cooker stoneware. Add broth.

2. Stir in squash and apples. Cover and cook on Low for 8 hours or on High for 4 hours, until squash is tender.

3. Preheat broiler. Working in batches, purée soup in a food processor or blender. (You can also do this in the stoneware using an immersion blender.) Ladle soup into ovenproof bowls. Sprinkle with cheese and broil until cheese melts, about 2 minutes. (You can also do this in a microwave oven, in batches, on High, about 1 minute per batch.) Sprinkle with walnuts, if using.

NUTRIENTS PER SERVING	
Calories	158
Fat	4.5 g
Saturates	1.7 g
Polyunsaturates	0.3 g
Monounsaturates	1.9 g
Cholesterol	9 mg
Sodium	329 mg
Carbohydrate	25.7 g
Fiber	4.1 g
Protein	6.2 g

AMERICA'S EXCHANGES	
1	Starch
2	Vegetable
1	Fat

CANADA'S CHOICES	
1½	Carbohydrate
½	Meat and Alternatives
½	Fat

MAKES 10 SERVINGS

Tip

To roast peppers: Preheat oven to 400°F (200°C). Place pepper(s) on a baking sheet and roast, turning two or three times, until the skin on all sides is blackened. (This will take about 25 minutes.) Transfer pepper(s) to a heatproof bowl. Cover with a plate and let stand until cool. Remove and, using a sharp knife, lift off skins. Discard skins, stem and core and slice according to recipe instructions.

Santa Fe Sweet Potato Soup

Here's a flavorful soup with lots of pizzazz and universal appeal. New Mexico chiles add an enticing, slightly smoky flavor, but ancho or guajillo chiles also work well. The lime, roasted red pepper and cilantro finish provides a nice balance to the sweet potatoes. If you are a heat seeker, add the jalapeño pepper.

- **Works best in a large (minimum 5 quart) slow cooker**

1 tbsp	olive oil	15 mL
2	onions, finely chopped	2
4	cloves garlic, minced	4
1 tsp	salt	5 mL
1 tsp	dried oregano leaves	5 mL
6 cups	lower-salt vegetable or chicken broth	1.5 L
4 cups	cubed peeled sweet potatoes (1/2-inch/1 cm cubes)	1 L
2	dried New Mexico, ancho or guajillo chile peppers	2
2 cups	boiling water	500 mL
1	jalapeño pepper, finely chopped, optional	1
2 cups	corn kernels, thawed if frozen	500 mL
1 tsp	grated lime zest	5 mL
2 tbsp	freshly squeezed lime juice	25 mL
2	roasted red peppers, cut into thin strips (see Tip, left)	2
	Finely chopped cilantro	

1. In a skillet, heat oil over medium heat for 30 seconds. Add onions and cook, stirring, until softened, about 3 minutes. Add garlic, salt and oregano and cook, stirring, for 1 minute. Transfer to slow cooker stoneware. Add broth and stir to combine.

2. Add sweet potatoes and stir to combine. Cover and cook on Low for 8 to 10 hours or on High for 4 to 6 hours, until sweet potatoes are tender.

NUTRIENTS PER SERVING	
Calories	157
Fat	2.4 g
Saturates	0.3 g
Polyunsaturates	0.5 g
Monounsaturates	1.1 g
Cholesterol	0 mg
Sodium	525 mg
Carbohydrate	32.4 g
Fiber	4.0 g
Protein	3.6 g

AMERICA'S EXCHANGES	
2	Starch

CANADA'S CHOICES	
2	Carbohydrate
1/2	Fat

This soup can be partially prepared before it is cooked. Complete Step 1. Cover and refrigerate for up to 2 days. When you're ready to cook, continue with the recipe.

3. Half an hour before soup has finished cooking, in a heatproof bowl, soak dried chile peppers in boiling water for 30 minutes, weighing down with a cup to ensure they remain submerged. Drain, discarding soaking liquid and stems. Pat dry, chop coarsely and add to stoneware, along with the jalapeño pepper, if using. Working in batches, purée soup in a food processor or blender and return to slow cooker. (You can also do this in the stoneware using an immersion blender.) Add corn, lime zest and juice. Cover and cook on High for 30 minutes, until corn is tender. When ready to serve, ladle soup into individual bowls and garnish with red pepper strips and cilantro.

Mindful Morsels

From mild and fruity to smoky and just plain fiery, chiles add depth as well as heat to any dish. Capsaicin is the substance that gives chiles their burn. Well known for causing a runny nose, chile peppers have long been used as a natural remedy for the congestion of a common cold. Capsaicin has also been found useful in treating certain types of pain; research into other uses, including disease prevention, is ongoing.

Vegetable Gumbo

This tasty vegetable soup reminds me of a delicious version of one of my favorite canned soups when I was a kid. Served with whole grain bread, it makes an excellent lunch.

Tips

This quantity of rice, combined with the okra, produces a dense soup, which condenses even more when refrigerated overnight. If you prefer a more soup-like consistency, add an additional cup (250 mL) of broth.

The brown rice in this recipe replaces the roux (flour cooked in oil) traditionally used to thicken gumbo. This reduces the quantity of fat and replaces refined flour with a healthy whole grain, adding fiber and other nutrients to the soup.

Okra, a traditional ingredient in gumbo, is a great thickener for broths, but be sure not to overcook it because it will become unpleasantly sticky. Choose young okra pods 2 to 4 inches (5 to 10 cm) long that don't feel sticky to the touch, in which case they are too ripe. Gently scrub the pods, cut off the top and tail and slice.

Make Ahead

This dish can be partially prepared before it is cooked. Complete Step 1. Cover and refrigerate overnight or for up to 2 days. When you're ready to cook, continue with Step 2.

- **Large (minimum 5 quart) slow cooker**

1 tbsp	olive oil	15 mL
2	onions, finely chopped	2
6	stalks celery, diced	6
4	cloves garlic, minced	4
2 tsp	dried thyme leaves, crumbled	10 mL
1/2 tsp	cracked black peppercorns	2 mL
1	bay leaf	1
1	can (28 oz/796 mL) diced tomatoes, including juice	1
1/2 cup	brown rice (see Tips, left)	125 mL
4 cups	Basic Vegetable Stock or Homemade Chicken Stock (see recipes, pages 38 and 39) or lower-salt broth	1 L
2 tsp	paprika, dissolved in 4 tsp (20 mL) lemon juice	10 mL
2 cups	sliced okra (1/4-inch/0.5 cm slices) (see Tips, left)	500 mL
1	green bell pepper, diced	1

1. In a skillet, heat oil over medium heat for 30 seconds. Add onions and celery and cook, stirring, until celery is softened, about 5 minutes. Add garlic, thyme, peppercorns and bay leaf and cook, stirring, for 1 minute. Add tomatoes with juice and bring to a boil. Transfer to slow cooker stoneware.

2. Add brown rice and stock. Cover and cook on Low for 6 hours or on High for 3 hours, until rice is tender. Discard bay leaf. Add paprika solution and stir well. Stir in okra and green pepper. Cover and cook on High for 20 minutes, until pepper is tender.

NUTRIENTS PER SERVING	
Calories	148
Fat	3.2 g
Saturates	0.5 g
Polyunsaturates	0.6 g
Monounsaturates	1.9 g
Cholesterol	0 mg
Sodium	238 mg
Carbohydrate	28.0 g
Fiber	4.7 g
Protein	4.5 g

AMERICA'S EXCHANGES	
1	Starch
2	Vegetable
1/2	Fat

CANADA'S CHOICES	
1 1/2	Carbohydrate
1/2	Fat

MAKES 8 SERVINGS

Tips

To toast cumin seeds: Place seeds in a dry skillet over medium heat, stirring, until fragrant, about 3 minutes. Immediately transfer to a mortar or a spice grinder and grind. If you prefer to use ground cumin, substitute half of the quantity called for.

In my opinion, cauliflower needs to be cooked quickly in rapidly boiling water. Cook it until it's tender to the bite, about 3 minutes after the water has returned to a boil, drain and add to the slow cooker.

Make Ahead

This soup can be partially prepared the night before it is cooked. Complete Step 1. Cover and refrigerate for up to 2 days. When you're ready to cook, continue with recipe.

Mulligatawny Soup

Mulligatawny, which means "pepper water" in Tamil, is an Anglo-Indian soup, imported to England by seafaring merchants. It is usually made with chicken, but a vegetarian version was documented by the great English cook Eliza Acton in her book Modern Cookery, published in 1845. This is a hearty and tasty soup that is suitable for many occasions, either as a first course or the focal point of a light meal.

- **Works best in a large (minimum 5 quart) slow cooker**

1 tbsp	olive oil	15 mL
2	onions, finely chopped	2
2	carrots, peeled and thinly sliced	2
4	stalks celery, thinly sliced	4
4	cloves garlic, minced	4
1 tsp	cumin seeds, toasted and ground (see Tips, left)	5 mL
1/2 tsp	salt	2 mL
1/2 tsp	cracked black peppercorns	2 mL
5 cups	lower-salt vegetable or chicken broth	1.25 L
2	medium potatoes, peeled and diced	2
1 tbsp	curry powder	15 mL
1 cup	low-fat plain yogurt, divided	250 mL
2 cups	cooked cauliflower florets (see Tips, left)	500 mL
	Finely chopped cilantro or parsley	

1. In a large skillet, heat oil over medium heat for 30 seconds. Add onions, carrots and celery and cook, stirring, until vegetables are softened, about 7 minutes. Add garlic, toasted cumin, salt and peppercorns and cook, stirring, for 1 minute. Transfer to slow cooker stoneware. Add broth and stir to combine.

2. Stir in potatoes. Cover and cook on Low for 8 to 10 hours or on High for 4 to 5 hours, until vegetables are tender. Working in batches, purée soup in a food processor or blender and return to slow cooker. (You can also do this in the stoneware using an immersion blender.)

3. In a small bowl, place curry powder. Gradually add 1/4 cup (50 mL) of the yogurt, beating until smooth. Add to stoneware along with remaining yogurt and cauliflower. Cover and cook on High for 30 minutes, until flavors meld. When ready to serve, ladle into bowls and garnish with cilantro.

NUTRIENTS PER SERVING	
Calories	102
Fat	2.7 g
Saturates	0.5 g
Polyunsaturates	0.3 g
Monounsaturates	1.4 g
Cholesterol	1 mg
Sodium	487 mg
Carbohydrate	16.5 g
Fiber	2.5 g
Protein	3.9 g

AMERICA'S EXCHANGES	
1/2	Starch
1 1/2	Vegetable
1/2	Fat

CANADA'S CHOICES	
1	Carbohydrate
1/2	Fat

Tips

To make crostini: Brush 10 baguette slices with olive oil on both sides. Toast under preheated broiler, turning once, until golden, about 2 minutes per side.

If you prefer a more pronounced garlic flavor, brush the baguette with garlic-infused oil.

If you don't have a mini-chopper, you can chop the roasted red pepper very finely and grate the garlic or put it through a press. Combine in a bowl with the mayonnaise and hot pepper sauce.

Bistro Fish Soup

Although it is described as soupe de poisson in France, where it is a mainstay of bistro culture, this ambrosial concoction is more closely related to a stew. It makes a satisfying main course accompanied by crusty rolls and a green salad.

- **Large (minimum 6 quart) slow cooker**

2 tbsp	olive oil	25 mL
3	large leeks, white part with a bit of green, cleaned and thinly sliced	3
1	onion, diced	1
1	bulb fennel, trimmed, cored and chopped, or 6 stalks celery, chopped	1
4	sprigs parsley or chervil	4
4	cloves garlic, minced	4
1 tsp	fennel seeds, crushed	5 mL
½ tsp	cracked black peppercorns	2 mL
1	can (28 oz/796 mL) diced tomatoes, including juice	1
6 cups	lower-salt vegetable broth	1.5 L
2 lbs	fish bones and pieces	1 kg
2	potatoes (about 1 lb/500 g), diced	2
1 tbsp	Pernod, optional	15 mL
½ cup	parsley leaves, finely chopped	125 mL
	Crostini (see Tips, left)	

Rouille

¼ cup	mayonnaise	50 mL
1	roasted red pepper, peeled and chopped	1
2	cloves garlic, minced	2
	Hot pepper sauce	
	Finely chopped parsley	

1. In a skillet, heat oil over medium heat for 30 seconds. Add leeks, onion and fennel and cook, stirring, until fennel is softened, about 6 minutes. Add parsley, garlic, fennel seeds and peppercorns and cook, stirring, for 1 minute. Add tomatoes, with juice, and broth and bring to a boil. Transfer to slow cooker stoneware.

NUTRIENTS PER SERVING	
Calories	220
Fat	9.7 g
Saturates	1.2 g
Polyunsaturates	2.2 g
Monounsaturates	5.8 g
Cholesterol	13 mg
Sodium	741 mg
Carbohydrate	26.4 g
Fiber	3.5 g
Protein	7.8 g

AMERICA'S EXCHANGES	
1½	Starch
2	Vegetable
2	Fat

CANADA'S CHOICES	
1½	Carbohydrate
½	Meat and Alternatives
1½	Fat

This recipe can be partially prepared before it is cooked. Complete Step 1. Cover and refrigerate overnight or for up to 2 days. When you're ready to cook, continue with Steps 2 and 3.

2. Add fish trimmings and potatoes and stir well. Cover and cook on Low for 8 to 10 hours or on High for 4 to 5 hours, until vegetables are very tender. Place a sieve over a large bowl or saucepan. Working in batches, ladle the soup into the sieve, removing and discarding any visible bones. Using a wooden spoon, push the solids through the sieve. Add Pernod, if using, to the strained soup. Add parsley and stir well.

3. **Rouille:** In a mini-chopper, combine mayonnaise, red pepper, garlic and hot pepper sauce to taste. Process until smooth. To serve, ladle hot soup into individual bowls and float a crostini on top of each serving. Garnish with parsley and top with a dollop of rouille.

Mindful Morsels

Along with garlic, leeks and onions belong to the Allium family. They are loaded with compounds containing sulfur, which is what makes your eyes water. But these compounds also seem to be associated with health benefits. There is limited evidence that eating onions on a regular basis raises beneficial high-density lipoproteins (HDL), lowers harmful triglycerides and lowers blood pressure. Be sure to include onions in the array of vegetables you eat. One-half cup (125 mL) of cooked onions contains about 11 g of carbohydrate, including 2 g of fiber.

Tips

To clean leeks: Fill a sink full of lukewarm water. Split the leeks in half lengthwise and submerge them in the water, swishing them around to remove all traces of dirt. Transfer to a colander and rinse thoroughly under cold water.

If you prefer, substitute 1 finely chopped fresh chile, such as jalapeño or cayenne, for the ground cayenne.

Make Ahead

This chowder can be partially prepared before it is cooked. Complete Steps 1 and 2. Cover and refrigerate for up to 2 days. When you're ready to cook, continue with the recipe.

Luscious Fish Chowder

This recipe makes a nicely peppery chowder, but if you're heat-averse, omit the cayenne. Although you can make an acceptable soup using water, clam juice or a good fish stock produce better results.

- **Works in slow cookers from 3½ to 6 quarts**

2	slices bacon, chopped	2
1 tbsp	olive oil	15 mL
3	leeks, white part only, cleaned and thinly sliced (see Tips, left)	3
3	stalks celery, thinly sliced	3
½ tsp	dried thyme leaves	2 mL
2 tbsp	all-purpose flour	25 mL
5 cups	fish stock or water or 2 cups (500 mL) bottled clam juice diluted with 3 cups (750 mL) water	1.25 L
1	bay leaf	1
1	medium potato, cut into ½-inch (1 cm) cubes	1
¼ tsp	cayenne pepper, or to taste (see Tips, left)	1 mL
1 cup	2% milk	250 mL
2 lbs	skinless firm white fish fillets, such as halibut or snapper, cut into 1-inch (2.5 cm) cubes	1 kg
	Finely chopped parsley or chives	

1. In a skillet, cook bacon over medium-high heat until crisp. Using a slotted spoon, remove and drain on paper towel. Cover and refrigerate until ready to use. Drain fat from pan. Add oil.

2. Reduce heat to medium. Add leeks and celery and cook, stirring, until softened, about 5 minutes. Stir in thyme and flour and cook, stirring, for 1 minute. Add stock and bay leaf. Bring to a boil and cook, stirring, until slightly thickened. Transfer mixture to slow cooker stoneware.

3. Add potato and stir. Cover and cook on Low for 8 to 10 hours or on High for 4 to 5 hours, until vegetables are tender.

4. Stir in cayenne. Add milk, fish and reserved bacon. Cover and cook on High for 30 minutes, or until fish is cooked through. Discard bay leaf. Ladle into individual bowls and garnish liberally with parsley.

NUTRIENTS PER SERVING	
Calories	164
Fat	4.7 g
Saturates	1.0 g
Polyunsaturates	1.0 g
Monounsaturates	2.1 g
Cholesterol	33 mg
Sodium	275 mg
Carbohydrate	9.0 g
Fiber	1.7 g
Protein	21.2 g

AMERICA'S EXCHANGES	
1½	Vegetable
3	Very Lean Meat

CANADA'S CHOICES	
½	Carbohydrate
3	Meat and Alternatives

Tips

Using the prunes will increase the Exchanges/Choices below by 1 Fruit/$\frac{1}{2}$ Carbohydrate.

If you're not using the prunes, add 1 cup (250 mL) additional lower-salt chicken broth along with the barley.

Although pearl barley is more readily available and tastes fine in this soup, make an effort to find whole (also known as hulled) barley when making the recipes in this book. It contains more nutrients, including fiber, than its refined relative. Pot barley, which is more refined than whole barley, is also a preferable alternative to pearl barley as it maintains some of the bran.

Make Ahead

This dish can be partially prepared before it is cooked. Complete Steps 1 through 3. Cover and refrigerate overnight or for up to 2 days. When you're ready to cook, continue with Step 4.

NUTRIENTS PER SERVING	
Calories	299
Fat	7.5 g
Saturates	1.7 g
Polyunsaturates	1.7 g
Monounsaturates	3.0 g
Cholesterol	109 mg
Sodium	166 mg
Carbohydrate	31.2 g
Fiber	5.1 g
Protein	27.2 g

Cockaleekie

This chicken and leek soup has been around for hundreds of years and qualifies as Scottish comfort food. Although the prunes seem unconventional, having tried the soup with and without this ingredient I prefer the addition of prunes, which add a pleasing sweetness and depth to the broth and complement the other flavors.

- **Large (minimum 6 quart) slow cooker**

20	pitted prunes, finely chopped (about 1 cup/ 250 mL) whole pitted prunes), optional (see Tip, left)	20
1½ cups	water	375 mL
2 lbs	boneless skinless chicken thighs	1 kg
1 tbsp	olive oil	15 mL
4	large leeks, white part with just a bit of green, cleaned and thinly sliced (see Tips, page 76)	4
4	stalks celery, diced	4
4	carrots, peeled and diced	4
1 tsp	dried thyme leaves, crumbled	5 mL
½ tsp	cracked black peppercorns	2 mL
4	whole cloves	4
1	piece (1 inch/2.5 cm) cinnamon stick	1
6 cups	Homemade Chicken Stock (see recipe, page 39) or lower-salt chicken broth	1.5 L
1 cup	whole (hulled) or pot barley, rinsed (see Tips, left)	250 mL
½ cup	finely chopped parsley	125 mL

1. In a small bowl, combine prunes and water. Stir well. Cover and set aside.

2. Arrange chicken over bottom of slow cooker stoneware.

3. In a large skillet, heat oil over medium heat for 30 seconds. Add leeks, celery and carrots and cook, stirring, until softened, about 7 minutes. Add thyme, peppercorns, cloves and cinnamon stick and cook, stirring for 1 minute. Transfer to slow cooker stoneware.

4. Add stock and barley. Cover and cook on Low for 6 hours or on High for 3 hours, until chicken is falling apart and barley is tender. Discard cloves and cinnamon stick. Add prunes and soaking water, if using. Stir well. Cover and cook on High for 30 minutes, until flavors have melded. Ladle into bowls and garnish with parsley.

AMERICA'S EXCHANGES	
1½	Starch
2	Vegetable
3	Very Lean Meat
½	Fat

CANADA'S CHOICES	
1½	Carbohydrate
3	Meat and Alternatives

Tips

You can also make this soup using cooked leftover turkey. Use 3 cups (750 mL) shredded turkey and add it along with the green pepper after the soup has cooked.

If you don't have pure ancho or New Mexico chili powder, use your favorite chili powder blend instead.

Add the jalapeño pepper if you like a bit of heat, or the chipotle pepper if you like a hint of smoke as well.

Turkey and Corn Chowder with Barley

A steaming bowl of this zesty, rib-sticking chowder will satisfy even the pickiest eater. It is equally good made with previously uncooked turkey or meat left over from the holiday bird. Add whole grain rolls and a green or sliced tomato salad for a delicious light meal.

- **Large (minimum 6 quart) slow cooker**

1 tbsp	cumin seeds	15 mL
1 tbsp	olive oil	15 mL
2	onions, finely chopped	2
6	stalks celery, diced	6
4	cloves garlic, minced	4
2 tsp	dried oregano leaves, crumbled	10 mL
½ tsp	cracked black peppercorns	2 mL
8 cups	Homemade Chicken Stock (see recipe, page 39) or lower-salt chicken or turkey broth	2 L
¾ cup	whole (hulled) or pot barley, rinsed	175 mL
2 lbs	skinless boneless turkey, cut into ½-inch (1 cm) cubes (about 3 cups/750 mL)	1 kg
2 cups	frozen corn kernels	500 mL
1 tsp	ancho or New Mexico chili powder, dissolved in 2 tbsp (25 mL) freshly squeezed lemon juice (see Tips, left)	5 mL
1	green bell pepper, seeded and diced	1
1	jalapeño pepper or chipotle pepper in adobo sauce, diced, optional (see Tips, left)	1
	Finely chopped cilantro, optional	

1. In a dry skillet over medium heat, toast cumin seeds, stirring, until fragrant and they just begin to brown, about 3 minutes. Immediately transfer to a mortar or a spice grinder and grind. Set aside.

2. In the same skillet, heat oil over medium heat for 30 seconds. Add onions and celery and cook, stirring, until celery is softened, about 5 minutes. Add garlic, oregano, peppercorns and reserved cumin and cook, stirring, for 1 minute. Transfer to slow cooker stoneware. Add stock and stir well.

NUTRIENTS PER SERVING

Calories	216
Fat	4.3 g
Saturates	1.0 g
Polyunsaturates	0.9 g
Monounsaturates	2.1 g
Cholesterol	56 mg
Sodium	97 mg
Carbohydrate	23.1 g
Fiber	2.8 g
Protein	22.3 g

AMERICA'S EXCHANGES	
1	Starch
1	Vegetable
2	Lean Meat

CANADA'S CHOICES	
1	Carbohydrate
2	Meat and Alternatives

Make Ahead

This dish can be partially prepared before it is cooked. Complete Steps 1 and 2. Cover and refrigerate overnight or for up to 2 days. When you're ready to cook, continue with Step 3.

3. Add barley, turkey and corn. Cover and cook on Low for 8 hours or on High for 4 hours, until turkey and barley are tender. Stir in chili powder solution. Add green pepper and jalapeño pepper, if using, and stir well. Cover and cook on High for 20 minutes, until pepper is tender. To serve, ladle into bowls and garnish with cilantro, if using.

Mindful Morsels

A serving of this tasty soup is an excellent source of vitamin B_6. The peppers and the turkey are a source of this important nutrient. Vitamin B_6 supports your nervous system, helping your body deal with stress, and also helps your body create the protein needed to make new cells.

Tips

To toast cumin seeds: Place seeds in a dry skillet over medium heat and cook, stirring, until fragrant and seeds just begin to brown, about 3 minutes. Immediately transfer to a mortar or a spice grinder and grind.

If you prefer a thicker, more integrated soup, purée the drained beans in a food processor or mash with a potato masher before adding to the stoneware.

You can also make this soup using cooked leftover turkey. Use 2½ cups (625 mL) of shredded turkey and add it along with the bell peppers.

If you don't have ancho chili powder, you can substitute an equal quantity of New Mexico chili powder, your favorite chili powder blend or ¼ tsp (1 mL) cayenne pepper.

Turkey and Black Bean Soup

This hearty soup is a meal in a bowl. I like to serve it with a simple green or shredded carrot salad and crusty whole grain bread for a great weeknight meal. The quantity of chili powder, combined with a chipotle pepper, produces a zesty result. If you're heat-averse, reduce the quantity of chili powder and use a jalapeño instead of a chipotle pepper.

• **Large (minimum 6 quart) slow cooker**

1 tbsp	olive oil	15 mL
2	onions, finely chopped	2
2	carrots, peeled and diced	2
2	stalks celery, diced	2
4	cloves garlic, minced	4
1 tbsp	dried oregano leaves, crumbled	15 mL
1 tsp	cracked black peppercorns	5 mL
1 tsp	finely grated lime zest	5 mL
2 tbsp	cumin seeds, toasted and ground (see Tips, left)	25 mL
¼ cup	tomato paste	50 mL
6 cups	Homemade Chicken Stock (see recipe, page 39) or lower-salt chicken broth	1.5 L
2	cans (each 14 oz/398 mL) black beans, drained and rinsed, or 3 cups (750 mL) cooked dried black beans (see Variation, page 231)	2
2½ cups	cubed (½ inch/1 cm) skinless boneless turkey breast (one 1½ lb/750 g bone-in turkey breast) (see Tips, left)	625 mL
2 tsp	ancho chili powder, dissolved in 2 tbsp (25 mL) freshly squeezed lime juice (see Tips, left)	10 mL
1	jalapeño pepper or chipotle pepper in adobo sauce, minced	1
1	green bell pepper, diced	1
1	red bell pepper, diced	1

NUTRIENTS PER SERVING	
Calories	231
Fat	4.8 g
Saturates	1.0 g
Polyunsaturates	1.0 g
Monounsaturates	2.4 g
Cholesterol	52 mg
Sodium	364 mg
Carbohydrate	23.6 g
Fiber	7.8 g
Protein	24.7 g

AMERICA'S EXCHANGES	
1	Starch
2	Vegetable
3	Very Lean Meat

CANADA'S CHOICES	
1	Carbohydrate
3	Meat and Alternatives

Make Ahead

This dish can be partially prepared before it is cooked. Complete Step 1. Cover and refrigerate overnight or for up to 2 days. When you're ready to cook, continue with Steps 2 and 3.

1. In a skillet, heat oil over medium heat for 30 seconds. Add onions, carrots and celery and cook, stirring, until softened, about 7 minutes. Add garlic, oregano, peppercorns, lime zest and toasted cumin and cook, stirring, for 1 minute. Add tomato paste and stir well. Transfer to slow cooker stoneware. Stir in stock and beans.

2. Add turkey and stir well. Cover and cook on Low for 6 hours or on High for 3 hours, until turkey is cooked and mixture is bubbly.

3. Add ancho solution and stir well. Add jalapeño and green and red bell peppers and stir well. Cover and cook on High for 20 minutes, until peppers are tender.

Mindful Morsels

One serving of this soup is an excellent source of vitamins A, C and B_6, potassium and iron. The slowly digested carbohydrate in beans helps stabilize blood glucose levels. It causes a smaller rise in blood glucose after meals than the same amount of carbohydrate from many other foods.

Scotch Broth

Tips

To clean leeks: Fill a sink full of lukewarm water. Split the leeks in half lengthwise and submerge them in the water, swishing them around to remove all traces of dirt. Transfer to a colander and rinse thoroughly under cold water.

Although pearl barley is more readily available, make an effort to find whole (also known as hulled) barley when making the recipes in this book. It contains more nutrients, including fiber, than its refined relative. Pot barley, which is more refined than whole barley, is also a preferable alternative to pearl barley as it maintains some of the bran.

Make Ahead

This dish can be partially prepared before it is cooked. Heat 1 tbsp (15 mL) oil and complete Step 2. Cover and refrigerate overnight or for up to 2 days. When you're ready to cook, either brown the lamb as outlined in Step 1 or add it to the stoneware without browning. Stir well and continue with Step 3.

This hearty meal-in-a bowl is known as Scotland's pot-au-feu, a traditional boiled dinner. It is usually made with lamb, but I have an old Scottish recipe that suggests beef or a "good marrow bone" may be substituted. I like to serve this as a light dinner, accompanied by a simple green salad and warm crusty rolls.

- **Large (minimum 6 quart) slow cooker**

1 tbsp	olive oil	15 mL
1 lb	lamb shoulder or stewing beef, trimmed of fat and diced	500 g
3	leeks, white and light green parts only, cleaned and thinly sliced (see Tips, left)	3
4	stalks celery, diced	4
4	carrots, peeled and diced	4
2	parsnips, peeled and diced	2
2 tsp	dried thyme leaves, crumbled	10 mL
1/2 tsp	cracked black peppercorns	2 mL
1	bay leaf	1
8 cups	lower-salt beef broth	2 L
1 cup	whole (hulled) or pot barley (see Tips, left), rinsed	250 mL
1 cup	green peas, thawed if frozen	250 mL
1/2 cup	finely chopped parsley leaves	125 mL

1. In a skillet, heat half the oil over medium-high heat for 30 seconds. Add lamb, in batches, and cook, stirring, adding remaining oil as necessary, until browned, about 1 minute per batch. Using a slotted spoon, transfer to slow cooker stoneware. Drain off fat.

2. Reduce heat to medium. Add leeks, celery, carrots and parsnips and cook, stirring, until vegetables are softened, about 7 minutes. Add thyme and peppercorns and cook, stirring, for 1 minute. Transfer to slow cooker stoneware. Stir in bay leaf and broth. Stir in barley.

3. Cover and cook on Low for 7 hours or on High for 3 1/2 hours, until vegetables are tender. Stir in green peas and cook on High for 20 minutes, until tender. Discard bay leaf. Serve hot, liberally garnished with parsley.

NUTRIENTS PER SERVING	
Calories	210
Fat	4.7 g
Saturates	1.2 g
Polyunsaturates	0.6 g
Monounsaturates	2.2 g
Cholesterol	26 mg
Sodium	465 mg
Carbohydrate	30.4 g
Fiber	4.9 g
Protein	13.0 g

AMERICA'S EXCHANGES	
2	Starch
1	Lean Meat

CANADA'S CHOICES	
1 1/2	Carbohydrate
1	Meat and Alternatives

Chilies

Vegetable Chili

MAKES 8 SERVINGS

Tips

If you don't have leeks, substitute 2 yellow onions, finely chopped.

If you prefer a more peppery chili, use up to 1 tsp (5 mL) of cracked black peppercorns in this recipe.

To toast cumin seeds: Place seeds in a dry skillet over medium heat and cook, stirring, until fragrant and seeds just begin to brown, about 3 minutes. Immediately transfer to a mortar or a spice grinder and grind.

You can substitute your favorite chili powder blend for the ancho or New Mexico chili powder.

Here's a chili that is loaded with flavor and nutrients. Garnish with any combination of roasted red peppers, diced avocado, finely chopped red onions and cilantro. Add a simple green salad and some whole grain bread for a great weekday meal.

- **Large (minimum 5 quart) slow cooker**

4 cups	thinly sliced zucchini (about 1 lb/500 g)	1 L
½ tsp	salt	2 mL
2 tbsp	olive oil, divided	25 mL
4	cloves garlic, minced	4
2	large leeks, white and green parts only, cleaned and thinly sliced (see Tips, left)	2
4	stalks celery, diced	4
4	carrots, peeled and diced	4
2 tsp	dried oregano leaves, crumbled	10 mL
½ tsp	cracked black peppercorns (see Tips, left)	2 mL
1 tbsp	cumin seeds, toasted and ground (see Tips, left)	15 mL
1	can (28 oz/796 mL) diced tomatoes, including juice	1
1	can (14 oz/398 mL) kidney or pinto beans, drained and rinsed	1
1 cup	bulgur	250 mL
1 tbsp	ancho or New Mexico chili powder, dissolved in 2 tbsp (25 mL) freshly squeezed lemon juice (see Tips, left)	15 mL
2	green bell peppers, diced	2
1	jalapeño or chipotle pepper in adobo sauce, diced	1
	Light sour cream, optional	

1. In a colander over a sink, combine zucchini and salt. Set aside to sweat for 20 minutes. Rinse thoroughly under cold running water and pat dry with paper towels. Set aside.

2. In a skillet, heat 1 tbsp (15 mL) of the oil over medium heat for 30 seconds. Add zucchini and cook, stirring, for 3 minutes. Add garlic and cook, stirring, until zucchini softens and just begins to brown, about 4 minutes. Transfer to a bowl, cover and refrigerate.

NUTRIENTS PER SERVING	
Calories	204
Fat	4.5 g
Saturates	0.6 g
Polyunsaturates	0.8 g
Monounsaturates	2.8 g
Cholesterol	0 mg
Sodium	480 mg
Carbohydrate	37.9 g
Fiber	9.3 g
Protein	7.2 g

AMERICA'S EXCHANGES	
2	Starch
2	Vegetable
½	Fat

CANADA'S CHOICES	
2	Carbohydrate
1	Fat

Make Ahead

This dish can be partially prepared before it is cooked. Complete Steps 1 through 3. Cover and refrigerate separately overnight or for up to 2 days. When you're ready to cook, continue with Steps 4 and 5.

3. In a skillet, heat remaining 1 tbsp (15 mL) of the oil over medium heat. Add leeks, celery and carrots and cook, stirring, until carrots are softened, about 7 minutes. Add oregano, peppercorns and toasted cumin and cook, stirring, for 1 minute. Add tomatoes with juice and bring to a boil. Transfer to stoneware.

4. Stir in beans. Cover and cook on Low for 6 hours or on High for 3 hours, until vegetables are tender.

5. In a bowl, combine bulgur and 1 cup (250 mL) boiling water. Set aside for 30 minutes, until water is absorbed. Meanwhile, add chili pepper solution to stoneware and stir well. Add bell peppers, jalapeño and reserved zucchini. Stir well. Cover and cook on High for 20 to 30 minutes, until peppers are tender. Stir in bulgur. Ladle chili into bowls and garnish each with 1 tbsp (15 mL) sour cream.

Mindful Morsels

One serving of this delicious chili provides more than 100% of the recommended daily intake (RDI) of vitamin A. Although vitamin A is famous for keeping your eyes healthy, it has other important functions, such as contributing to your night-vision capabilities, supporting bone growth and keeping cells functioning well.

Light Chili

This is my favorite light chili. I love the rich, creamy sauce and the flavors of the spices. Serve this with a dab of light sour cream, your favorite salsa and a sprinkling of chopped cilantro.

MAKES 6 SERVINGS

• **Works in slow cookers from 3½ to 6 quarts**

1 tbsp	olive oil	15 mL
2	onions, finely chopped	2
6	cloves garlic, minced	6
1 tbsp	cumin seeds, toasted and ground (see Tips, left)	15 mL
1 tbsp	dried oregano leaves	15 mL
½ tsp	salt	2 mL
1 tsp	cracked black peppercorns	5 mL
1	can (28 oz/796 mL) diced tomatoes, including juice (see Tips, left)	1
2 cups	lower-salt vegetable broth	500 mL
8 oz	portobello mushrooms, stems removed, caps cut into 1-inch (2.5 cm) cubes	250 g
1	can (19 oz/540 mL) white kidney beans, drained and rinsed	1
1 to 2	jalapeño peppers, finely chopped	1 to 2
2	green bell peppers, diced	2
1½ cups	shredded light Monterey Jack cheese	375 mL
1	can (4½ oz/127 mL) diced mild green chiles, drained	1
	Salsa	
	Finely chopped cilantro	

Tips

To toast cumin seeds: Place seeds in a dry skillet over medium heat and cook, stirring, until fragrant and seeds just begin to brown, about 3 minutes. Immediately transfer to a mortar or a spice grinder and grind.

Large cans of tomatoes come in 28 oz (796 mL) and 35 oz (980 mL) sizes. For convenience, I've called for the 28 oz (796 mL) size in my recipes. If you're using the 35 oz (980 mL) size, drain off 1 cup (250 mL) liquid before adding to the recipe.

Make Ahead

This dish can be partially prepared before it is cooked. Chop jalapeño and bell peppers and shred cheese. Cover and refrigerate. Complete Step 1. Cover and refrigerate for up to 2 days. When you're ready to cook, continue with the recipe.

1. In a skillet, heat oil over medium heat for 30 seconds. Add onions and cook, stirring, until softened, about 3 minutes. Add garlic, toasted cumin, oregano, salt and peppercorns and cook, stirring, for 1 minute. Add tomatoes, with juice, and broth and bring to a boil. Cook, stirring, until liquid is reduced by one-third, about 5 minutes. Transfer to slow cooker stoneware.

2. Add mushrooms and beans and stir to combine. Cover and cook on Low for 6 to 8 hours or on High for 3 to 4 hours, until mixture is hot and bubbly. Stir in jalapeño peppers, green peppers, cheese and mild green chiles. Cover and cook on High for 20 to 30 minutes, until peppers are tender and cheese is melted. Ladle into bowls and top with salsa and chopped cilantro.

NUTRIENTS PER SERVING	
Calories	274
Fat	9.8 g
Saturates	4.4 g
Polyunsaturates	0.9 g
Monounsaturates	3.4 g
Cholesterol	18 mg
Sodium	586 mg
Carbohydrate	32.7 g
Fiber	10.0 g
Protein	16.9 g

AMERICA'S EXCHANGES	
2	Starch
2	Lean Meat

CANADA'S CHOICES	
1½	Carbohydrate
2	Meat and Alternatives

Tips

To toast cumin seeds: Place seeds in a dry skillet over medium heat and cook, stirring, until fragrant and seeds just begin to brown, about 3 minutes. Immediately transfer to a mortar or a spice grinder and grind.

Add the chipotle pepper if you like heat and a bit of smoke.

Make Ahead

This dish can be partially prepared before it is cooked. Complete Step 1. Cover and refrigerate overnight or for up to 2 days. When you're ready to cook, continue with Step 2.

Squash and Black Bean Chili

Flavored with cumin and chili powder, with a hint of cinnamon, this luscious chili makes a fabulous weeknight meal. Add a tossed green salad and a whole grain roll, relax and enjoy.

- **Works in slow cookers from 3½ to 6 quarts**

1 tbsp	olive oil	15 mL
2	onions, finely chopped	2
4	cloves garlic, minced	4
2 tsp	chili powder	10 mL
1 tsp	dried oregano leaves	5 mL
1 tsp	cumin seeds, toasted (see Tips, left)	5 mL
1	piece (3 inches/7.5 cm) cinnamon stick	1
1	can (28 oz/796 mL) diced tomatoes, including juice	1
1	can (14 to 19 oz/398 to 540 mL) black beans, drained and rinsed, or 1 cup (250 mL) dried black beans, soaked, cooked and drained (see Variation, page 231)	1
4 cups	cubed (1 inch/2.5 cm) peeled butternut squash	1 L
2	green bell peppers, diced	2
1	can (4½ oz/127 mL) chopped mild green chiles	1
1	finely chopped chipotle pepper in adobo sauce, optional	1
	Finely chopped fresh cilantro leaves	

1. In a skillet, heat oil over medium heat for 30 seconds. Add onions to pan and cook, stirring, until softened, about 3 minutes. Add garlic, chili powder, oregano, toasted cumin and cinnamon stick and cook, stirring, for 1 minute. Add tomatoes with juice and bring to a boil. Transfer to slow cooker stoneware. Add beans and squash and stir well.

2. Cover and cook on Low for 8 hours or on High for 4 hours, until squash is tender. Add bell peppers, chiles and chipotle pepper, if using. Cover and cook on High for 20 minutes, until bell pepper is tender. Discard cinnamon stick. When ready to serve, ladle into bowls and garnish with cilantro.

NUTRIENTS PER SERVING	
Calories	171
Fat	3.1 g
Saturates	0.4 g
Polyunsaturates	0.6 g
Monounsaturates	1.8 g
Cholesterol	0 mg
Sodium	589 mg
Carbohydrate	33.5 g
Fiber	8.1 g
Protein	6.6 g

AMERICA'S EXCHANGES	
1½	Starch
2	Vegetable

CANADA'S CHOICES	
1½	Carbohydrate
1	Meat and Alternatives

MAKES 6 SERVINGS

Tips

Use your favorite chili powder blend in this recipe or, if you prefer, ground ancho, New Mexico or guajillo peppers.

I prefer the slightly smoky flavor that a chipotle pepper in adobo sauce lends to this recipe, but it's not to everyone's taste. If you're unfamiliar with the flavor, add just half a pepper and a bit of the sauce. If you're a heat seeker, use a whole one and increase the quantity of adobo sauce.

Barley and Sweet Potato Chili

This unusual chili has great flavor and with the addition of optional toppings, such as sliced roasted pepper strips (either bottled or freshly roasted) and cilantro, it can be enhanced and varied to suit many tastes. I like to serve this with a simple green salad topped with sliced avocado.

• **Large (minimum 5 quart) slow cooker**

1 tbsp	cumin seeds	15 mL
1 tbsp	olive oil	15 mL
2	onions, finely chopped	2
2	cloves garlic, minced	2
1 tsp	dried oregano leaves, crumbled	5 mL
½ tsp	salt	2 mL
½ tsp	cracked black peppercorns	2 mL
½ cup	whole (hulled) or pot barley	125 mL
1	can (28 oz/796 mL) tomatoes, including juice, coarsely crushed	1
1 cup	lower-salt vegetable broth	250 mL
2	medium sweet potatoes, peeled and cut into 1-inch (2.5 cm) cubes	2
1	can (14 to 19 oz/398 to 540 mL) red kidney or black beans, drained and rinsed, or 1 cup (250 mL) dried red kidney or black beans, soaked, cooked and drained (see Variation, page 231)	1
1 tbsp	chili powder, dissolved in 2 tbsp (25 mL) lime juice (see Tips, left)	15 mL
1	jalapeño pepper, minced, or ½ to 1 chipotle pepper in adobo sauce, minced (see Tips, left)	1
1	green bell pepper, diced, optional	1
	Sliced roasted bell peppers, optional	
	Finely chopped cilantro	

1. In a large dry skillet over medium heat, toast cumin seeds, stirring, until fragrant and they just begin to brown, about 3 minutes. Immediately transfer to a mortar or spice grinder and grind. Set aside.

NUTRIENTS PER SERVING	
Calories	217
Fat	3.4 g
Saturates	0.5 g
Polyunsaturates	0.7 g
Monounsaturates	1.9 g
Cholesterol	0 mg
Sodium	636 mg
Carbohydrate	42.6 g
Fiber	7.3 g
Protein	6.5 g

AMERICA'S EXCHANGES	
2	Starch
2	Vegetable

CANADA'S CHOICES	
2	Carbohydrate
½	Fat

Make Ahead

This dish can be partially prepared before it is cooked. Complete Steps 1 and 2. Cover and refrigerate overnight or for up to 2 days. When you're ready to cook, continue with Step 3.

2. In same skillet, heat oil over medium heat for 30 seconds. Add onions and cook, stirring, until softened, about 3 minutes. Add garlic, oregano, salt, peppercorns and reserved cumin and cook, stirring, for 1 minute. Add barley and stir well. Add tomatoes with juice and bring to a boil. Transfer to slow cooker stoneware. Add broth, sweet potatoes and beans.

3. Cover and cook on Low for 6 to 8 hours or on High for 3 to 4 hours, until barley and sweet potatoes are tender. Stir in chili powder solution, jalapeño pepper and green pepper, if using. Cover and cook on High for 20 to 30 minutes, until flavors have melded and green pepper is tender. To serve, ladle into soup plates and garnish with roasted pepper strips, if using, and cilantro.

Mindful Morsels

The nutrient analysis on this recipe was done using pearl barley. For added fiber and nutrients, look for whole (also known as hulled) barley.

Brown Rice Chili

MAKES 10 SERVINGS

This tasty chili is an ideal dish for vegetarians as the combination of rice and beans produces a complete protein. I think the flavor is outstanding when it's made using reconstituted dried chiles. Just be aware that chiles described as New Mexico can range widely in heat. If you are using New Mexico chiles in this recipe, check to make certain that they are not described as "hot." The "mild" variety is called for.

Tip

Large cans of tomatoes come in 28 oz (796 mL) and 35 oz (980 mL) sizes. For convenience, I've called for the 28 oz (796 mL) size in my recipes. If you're using the 35 oz (980 mL) size, drain off 1 cup (250 mL) liquid before adding to the recipe.

• **Works best in a large (minimum 5 quart) slow cooker**

1 tbsp	olive oil	15 mL
2	onions, chopped	2
4	stalks celery, chopped	4
1 cup	brown rice, rinsed	250 mL
4	cloves garlic, finely chopped	4
1 tbsp	dried oregano leaves	15 mL
1 tsp	ground cumin	5 mL
½ tsp	salt	2 mL
½ tsp	cracked black peppercorns	2 mL
1	can (28 oz/796 mL) diced tomatoes, including juice (see Tip, left)	1
2 cups	cooked dried or canned red kidney beans, drained and rinsed	500 mL
2 cups	lower-salt vegetable broth, divided	500 mL
2	dried ancho, mild New Mexico or guajillo chile peppers	2
2 cups	boiling water	500 mL
½ cup	chopped cilantro stems and leaves	125 mL
2 cups	corn kernels, thawed if frozen	500 mL
1	green bell pepper, diced	1
1	jalapeño pepper, seeded and diced, optional	1

1. In a skillet, heat oil over medium heat for 30 seconds. Add onions and celery and cook, stirring, until celery is softened, about 5 minutes. Add rice, garlic, oregano, cumin, salt and peppercorns and cook, stirring, for 1 minute. Add tomatoes with juice and bring to a boil. Transfer to slow cooker stoneware. Add beans and 1½ cups (375 mL) of the broth and stir well.

NUTRIENTS PER SERVING	
Calories	206
Fat	3.0 g
Saturates	0.4 g
Polyunsaturates	0.8 g
Monounsaturates	1.3 g
Cholesterol	0 mg
Sodium	479 mg
Carbohydrate	39.9 g
Fiber	7.7 g
Protein	7.7 g

AMERICA'S EXCHANGES	
2½	Starch

CANADA'S CHOICES	
2	Carbohydrate
½	Meat and Alternatives

Make Ahead

This dish can be partially prepared before it is cooked. Complete Steps 1 and 3. Cover and refrigerate onion and chile mixtures separately, overnight. (For best results, rehydrate chiles while the chili is cooking.) When you're ready to cook, continue with the recipe.

2. Place two clean tea towels, each folded in half (so you will have four layers) over top of stoneware. Cover and cook on Low for 8 hours or on High for 4 hours, until hot and bubbly.

3. Half an hour before recipe has finished cooking, in a heatproof bowl, soak chile peppers in boiling water for 30 minutes, weighing down with a cup to ensure they remain submerged. Drain, discarding soaking water and stems, and chop coarsely. Transfer to a blender. Add remaining broth and cilantro. Purée.

4. Add chile mixture, corn, bell pepper and jalapeño pepper, if using, to stoneware and stir well. Cover and cook on High for 30 minutes, until pepper is tender and flavors meld.

Mindful Morsels

Low in calories, tomatoes are extremely nutritious. They contain vitamins A and C, potassium and folacin and are loaded with phytonutrients such as lycopene, a powerful antioxidant that may have cancer-fighting properties.

Tamale Pie with Chili Millet Crust

MAKES 10 SERVINGS

Tips

To toast cumin seeds: Place seeds in a skillet over medium heat, stirring, until fragrant and they just begin to brown, about 3 minutes. Immediately transfer to a mortar or spice grinder and grind.

If you don't care for much heat, use the jalapeño pepper. Heat seekers may prefer a whole chipotle in adobo sauce.

This tasty pie is a great dish for après ski or to come home to after a brisk day outdoors. Add a tossed green salad, and pass the salsa at the table.

- **Large (minimum 6 quart) slow cooker**

1 tbsp	olive oil	15 mL
2	onions, finely chopped	2
4	stalks celery, thinly sliced	4
4	cloves garlic, minced	4
2 tsp	dried oregano leaves, crumbled	10 mL
1 tsp	salt	5 mL
1/2 tsp	cracked black peppercorns	2 mL
1 tbsp	cumin seeds, toasted and ground (see Tips, left)	15 mL
2	cans (each 14 oz/398 mL) black or pinto beans, drained and rinsed	2
1	can (28 oz/796 mL) diced tomatoes, drained	1
2 cups	frozen corn kernels	500 mL
1	green bell pepper, diced	1
1	jalapeño pepper or chipotle pepper in adobo sauce, diced (see Tips, left)	1
	Salsa, optional	

Topping

1 cup	millet	250 mL
3 cups	water	750 mL
	Freshly ground black pepper	
1 cup	shredded light Monterey Jack cheese	250 mL
1	can (4 1/2 oz/127 mL) chopped mild green chiles, including juice	1

1. In a skillet, heat oil over medium heat for 30 seconds. Add onions and celery and cook, stirring, until celery is softened, about 5 minutes. Add garlic, oregano, salt, peppercorns and toasted cumin and cook, stirring, for 1 minute. Add beans and tomatoes and bring to a boil. Transfer to stoneware.

NUTRIENTS PER SERVING	
Calories	235
Fat	4.6 g
Saturates	1.4 g
Polyunsaturates	0.8 g
Monounsaturates	1.8 g
Cholesterol	6 mg
Sodium	665 mg
Carbohydrate	39 g
Fiber	8.3 g
Protein	11.6 g

AMERICA'S EXCHANGES	
2	Starch
2	Vegetable
1	Very Lean Meat
1	Fat

CANADA'S CHOICES	
2	Carbohydrate
1	Meat and Alternatives

Make Ahead

This dish can be partially prepared before it is cooked. Complete Step 1. Cover and refrigerate overnight or for up to 2 days. When you're ready to cook, continue with Steps 2 through 4.

2. Add corn and stir well. Cover and cook on Low for 3 hours or on High for $1\frac{1}{2}$ hours.

3. **Topping:** In a saucepan over medium heat, toast millet, stirring constantly, until it crackles and releases its aroma, about 5 minutes. Add water and black pepper to taste, and bring to a boil. Reduce heat to low, cover and cook until millet is tender and all of the water is absorbed, about 20 minutes. Stir in cheese and chiles with juice and set aside.

4. Add bell pepper and jalapeño pepper to slow cooker stoneware and stir well. Spread millet topping evenly over pie. Place two clean tea towels, each folded in half (so you will have four layers) over top of stoneware to absorb moisture. Cover and cook on High for $1\frac{1}{2}$ to 2 hours, until topping is set.

Mindful Morsels

A serving of this recipe provides folacin, a B vitamin essential for the proper development of all cells in the body. Good sources of naturally occurring folacin are dried peas and beans, orange juice, and vegetables such as broccoli, asparagus, green beans and tomatoes.

Chili con Carne

Because it contains beans, this chili doesn't qualify as a "Texas" version, but in my opinion, it is every bit as flavorful. It is also much more nutritious because it balances the quantity of red meat with other healthful ingredients such as onions, garlic, peppers, kidney beans, cumin and oregano. Add a nutrient-dense garnish, such as strips of roasted red pepper, and be sure to keep the sour cream in check.

To toast cumin seeds: Place seeds in a dry skillet over medium heat and cook, stirring, until fragrant and seeds just begin to brown, about 3 minutes. Immediately transfer to a mortar or a spice grinder and grind.

I've provided a range of fresh peppers in this recipe so you can select to suit your taste and their availability. The poblano and Anaheim chiles are mildly hot. Green bell peppers produce a milder, but equally pleasant chili.

- **Works in slow cookers from 3½ to 6 quarts**

⅓ cup	all-purpose flour	75 mL
1 tsp	salt	5 mL
2 lbs	trimmed stewing beef, cut into 1-inch (2.5 cm) cubes	1 kg
2 tbsp	olive oil, divided (approx.)	25 mL
2	onions, finely chopped	2
4	cloves garlic, minced	4
1 tbsp	dried oregano leaves, crumbled	15 mL
1	piece (2 inches/5 cm) cinnamon stick	1
1 tsp	cracked black peppercorns	5 mL
2 tbsp	cumin seeds, toasted and ground (see Tips, left)	25 mL
1 cup	lower-salt beef broth	250 mL
1 cup	lager or pilsner beer	250 mL
2	cans (each 14 to 19 oz/398 to 540 mL) red kidney beans, rinsed and drained, or 2 cups (500 mL) dried red kidney beans, soaked, cooked and drained (see Variation, page 231)	2
1 tbsp	ancho chili powder or ½ tsp (2 mL) cayenne, dissolved in 2 tbsp (25 mL) lime juice	15 mL
1	jalapeño pepper or chipotle pepper in adobo sauce, minced	1
2	poblano or Anaheim chiles or green bell peppers, diced (see Tips, left)	2
	Finely chopped cilantro	
	Sour cream	
	Chopped red onion	
	Roasted red pepper strips	

NUTRIENTS PER SERVING	
Calories	263
Fat	9.0 g
Saturates	2.5 g
Polyunsaturates	0.8 g
Monounsaturates	4.1 g
Cholesterol	38 mg
Sodium	580 mg
Carbohydrate	22.1 g
Fiber	6.5 g
Protein	23.5 g

AMERICA'S EXCHANGES	
1½	Starch
2½	Lean Meat

CANADA'S CHOICES	
1	Carbohydrate
3	Meat and Alternatives

Make Ahead

This dish can be partially prepared before it is cooked. Heat 1 tbsp (15 mL) of the oil and complete Step 2. Cover and refrigerate overnight or for up to 2 days. When you're ready to cook, brown the beef as outlined in Step 1. Stir well and continue with Step 3.

1. In a resealable plastic bag, combine flour and salt. Add beef and toss until evenly coated, discarding excess flour mixture. In a skillet, heat 1 tbsp (15 mL) of the oil over medium-high heat for 30 seconds. Add beef, in batches, and cook, stirring, adding more oil as necessary, until browned, about 4 minutes per batch. Transfer to slow cooker stoneware.

2. Reduce heat to medium. Add onions to pan and cook, stirring, until softened, about 3 minutes. Add garlic, oregano, cinnamon stick, peppercorns and toasted cumin and cook, stirring, for 1 minute. Add broth and bring to a boil. Transfer to slow cooker stoneware. Add beer and beans and stir well.

3. Cover and cook on Low for 8 to 10 hours or on High for 4 to 5 hours, until beef is tender. Add chili powder solution, jalapeño pepper and poblano peppers and stir well. Cover and cook on High for 20 minutes, until fresh peppers are tender. Discard cinnamon stick. Serve with garnishes of your choice.

Mindful Morsels

You can reduce the amount of sodium in this dish by using canned beans with no salt added or cooking dried beans from scratch or reducing the quantity of salt used to flavor the beef.

Tip

If you prefer, you can soak and purée the chiles while preparing the chili and refrigerate until you're ready to add them to the recipe.

Make Ahead

This dish can be partially prepared before it is cooked. Complete Steps 1 and 3. Cover and refrigerate tomato and chile mixtures separately overnight. The next morning, continue with the recipe.

Butternut Chili

I love this chili. The combination of beef, butternut squash, ancho chiles and cilantro is a real winner. Don't be afraid to make extra, because it's great reheated.

- **Large (minimum 5 quart) slow cooker**

1 tbsp	olive oil	15 mL
1 lb	lean ground beef	500 g
2	onions, finely chopped	2
4	cloves garlic, minced	4
1 tbsp	cumin seeds, toasted and ground (see Tips, page 98)	15 mL
2 tsp	dried oregano leaves	10 mL
1 tsp	salt	5 mL
1/2 tsp	cracked black peppercorns	2 mL
1	piece (2 inches/5 cm) cinnamon stick	1
1	can (28 oz/796 mL) diced tomatoes, including juice	1
3 cups	cubed (1 inch/2.5 cm) peeled butternut squash	750 mL
2 cups	cooked dried or canned kidney beans, drained and rinsed	500 mL
2	dried New Mexico, ancho or guajillo chiles	2
2 cups	boiling water	500 mL
1/2 cup	coarsely chopped cilantro	125 mL

1. In a skillet, heat oil over medium-high heat for 30 seconds. Add beef and onions and cook, stirring, until beef is no longer pink, about 5 minutes. Add garlic, toasted cumin, oregano, salt, peppercorns and cinnamon stick and cook, stirring, for 1 minute. Add diced tomatoes with juice and bring to a boil.

2. Place squash and beans in slow cooker stoneware and cover with sauce. Cover and cook on Low for 6 to 8 hours or on High for 3 to 4 hours, until squash is tender.

3. Half an hour before recipe is finished cooking, in a heatproof bowl, soak dried chile peppers in boiling water for 30 minutes, weighing down with a cup to ensure they are submerged. Drain, reserving 1/2 cup (125 mL) of the soaking liquid. Discard stems and chop coarsely. In a blender, combine rehydrated chiles, cilantro and reserved soaking liquid. Purée. Add to stoneware and stir well. Cover and Cook on High for 30 minutes, until hot and bubbly and flavors meld.

NUTRIENTS PER SERVING	
Calories	270
Fat	10.6 g
Saturates	3.5 g
Polyunsaturates	0.9 g
Monounsaturates	4.8 g
Cholesterol	34 mg
Sodium	654 mg
Carbohydrate	28.2 g
Fiber	8.2 g
Protein	17.9 g

AMERICA'S EXCHANGES	
2	Starch
3	Lean Meat
1	Fat

CANADA'S CHOICES	
1 1/2	Carbohydrate
3	Meat and Alternatives
1	Fat

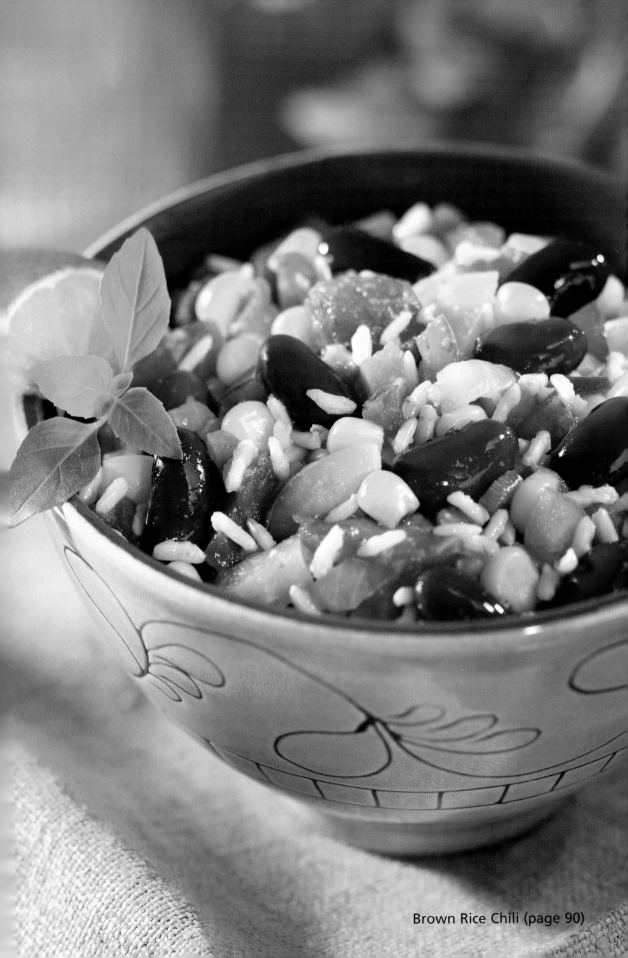

Brown Rice Chili (page 90)

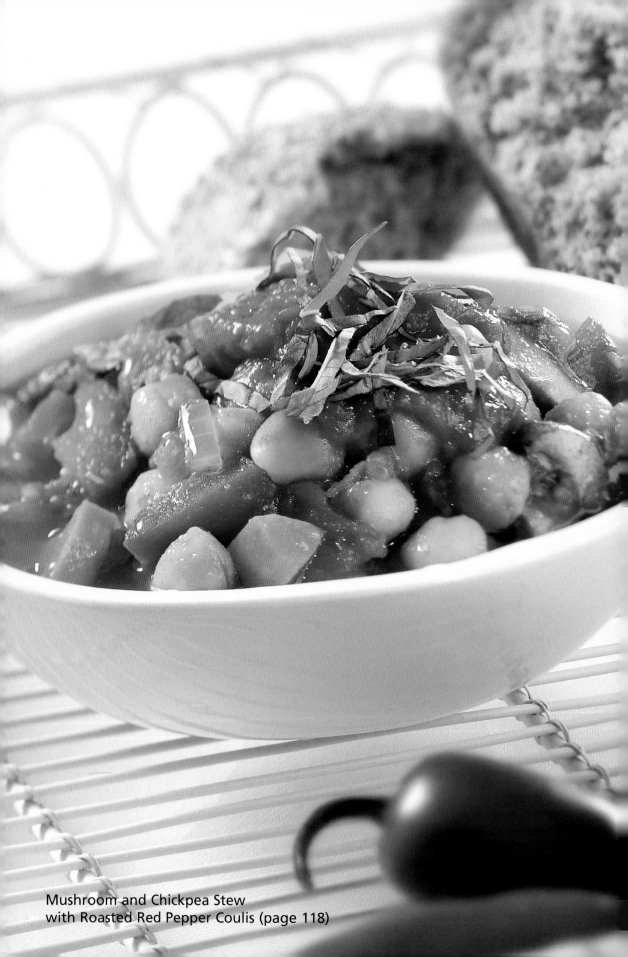

Mushroom and Chickpea Stew
with Roasted Red Pepper Coulis (page 118)

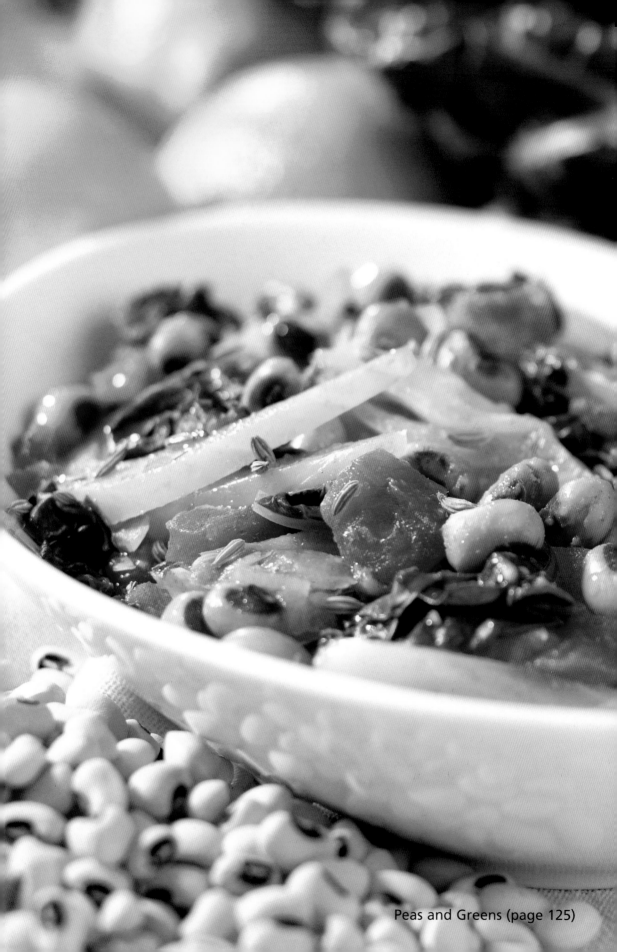

Peas and Greens (page 125)

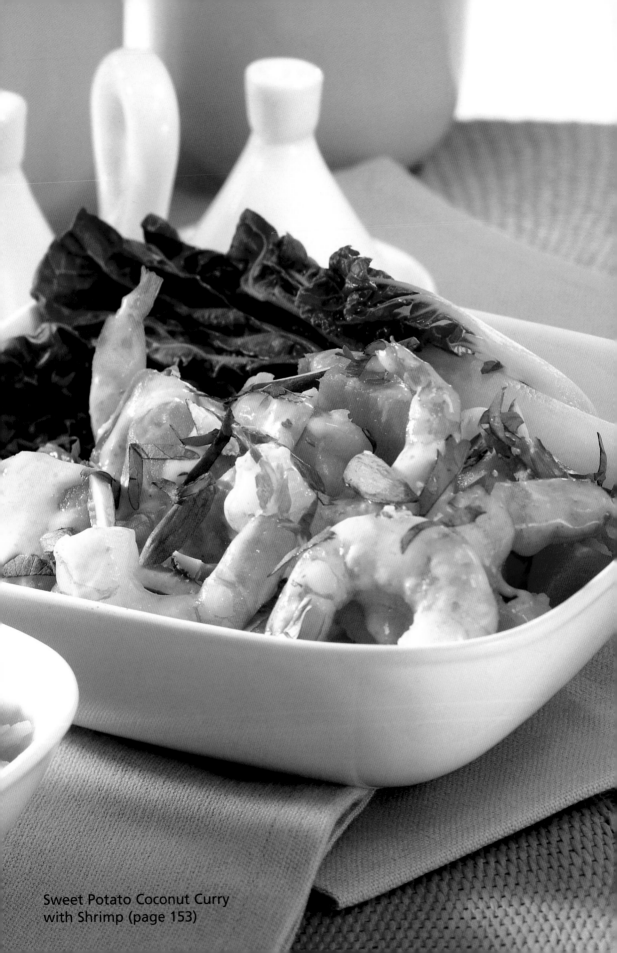

Sweet Potato Coconut Curry
with Shrimp (page 153)

Chunky Black Bean Chili

Here is a great-tasting, stick-to-the-ribs chili that is perfect for a family dinner or casual evening with friends.

Make Ahead

This dish can be partially prepared before it is cooked. Complete Steps 2 and 4, heating 1 tbsp (15 mL) oil in pan before softening the onions. Cover and refrigerate tomato and chile mixtures separately for up to 2 days, being aware that chile mixture will lose some of its vibrancy if held for this long. (For best results, rehydrate chiles while the chili is cooking or no sooner than the night before you plan to cook.) When you're ready to cook, brown the beef, or if you're pressed for time, omit this step. Continue with the recipe.

- **Large (minimum 5 quart) slow cooker**

1 tbsp	olive oil	15 mL
2 lbs	trimmed stewing beef, cut into 1-inch (2.5 cm) cubes	1 kg
2	onions, finely chopped	2
4	cloves garlic, minced	4
1 tbsp	cumin seeds, toasted and ground	15 mL
1 tbsp	dried oregano leaves, crumbled	15 mL
1 tsp	each cracked black peppercorns and salt	5 mL
1	can (28 oz/796 mL) diced tomatoes, including juice	1
1½ cups	flat beer or lower-salt beef broth, divided	375 mL
4 cups	cooked black beans, drained and rinsed	1 L
2	each dried ancho and New Mexico chile peppers	2
1 cup	coarsely chopped cilantro, leaves and stems	250 mL
1 to 2	jalapeño peppers, chopped, optional	1 to 2

1. In a skillet, heat oil over medium-high heat for 30 seconds. Add beef, in batches, and cook, stirring, adding a bit more oil if necessary, until lightly browned, about 4 minutes per batch. Using a slotted spoon, transfer to stoneware.

2. Reduce heat to medium. Add onions and cook, stirring, until softened. Add garlic, cumin, oregano, peppercorns and salt and cook, stirring, for 1 minute. Add tomatoes with juice and cook, breaking up with the back of a spoon, until desired consistency is achieved. Add 1 cup (250 mL) of the beer and bring to a boil.

3. Pour mixture over beef. Add beans and stir well. Cover and cook on Low for 8 to 10 hours or on High for 4 to 5 hours, until beef is tender.

4. Half an hour before recipe is finished cooking, in a heatproof bowl, soak ancho and New Mexico chiles in 4 cups (1 L) boiling water for 30 minutes, weighing down with a cup to ensure they remain submerged. Drain, discarding soaking liquid and stems, and chop coarsely. Transfer to a blender. Add cilantro, jalapeño, if using, and remaining beer. Purée.

5. Add chile mixture to stoneware and stir well. Cover and cook on High for 30 minutes, until mixture is hot and bubbly and flavors meld.

NUTRIENTS PER SERVING	
Calories	223
Fat	7.6 g
Saturates	2.3 g
Polyunsaturates	0.7 g
Monounsaturates	3.1 g
Cholesterol	38 mg
Sodium	534 mg
Carbohydrate	17.1 g
Fiber	4.4 g
Protein	21.6 g

AMERICA'S EXCHANGES	
1	Starch
3	Lean Meat

CANADA'S CHOICES	
1	Carbohydrate
3	Meat and Alternatives

Pork and Black Bean Chili

Tips

To toast cumin seeds: Place seeds in a dry skillet over medium heat and cook, stirring, until fragrant and seeds just begin to brown, about 3 minutes. Immediately transfer to a mortar or a spice grinder and grind.

Count 1 tbsp (15 mL) light sour cream as a Free Food/Extra.

Here's a festive and stick-to-your-ribs chili that is a perfect finish to a day in the chilly outdoors. I like to serve this with hot corn bread, a crisp green salad and a robust red wine or ice cold beer. Olé!

• **Works best in a large (minimum 5 quart) slow cooker**

1 tbsp	olive oil	15 mL
2 lbs	trimmed boneless pork shoulder, cut into 1-inch (2.5 cm) cubes, patted dry	1 kg
2	onions, finely chopped	2
4	cloves garlic, minced	4
1 tbsp	cumin seeds, toasted and ground (see Tips, left)	15 mL
1 tbsp	dried oregano leaves	15 mL
1 tsp	salt	5 mL
½ tsp	cracked black peppercorns	2 mL
2 tbsp	tomato paste	25 mL
1½ cups	flat beer	375 mL
4 cups	cooked dried or canned black beans, drained and rinsed (see Variation, page 231)	1 L
2	dried ancho chile peppers	2
2 cups	boiling water	500 mL
1 cup	coarsely chopped cilantro, stems and leaves	250 mL
½ cup	lower-salt chicken broth	125 mL
1	chipotle pepper in adobo sauce	1
	Light sour cream, optional	
	Finely chopped red or green onion, optional	

1. In a skillet, heat half the oil over medium-high heat for 30 seconds. Add pork, in batches, and cook, stirring, adding remaining oil as necessary, until browned, about 4 minutes per batch. Using a slotted spoon, transfer to stoneware.

2. Reduce heat to medium. Add onions to pan and cook, stirring, until softened, about 3 minutes. Add garlic, toasted cumin, oregano, salt and peppercorns and cook, stirring, for 1 minute. Stir in tomato paste and beer.

3. Pour mixture over meat. Add beans and stir to combine. Cover and cook on Low for 8 hours or on High for 4 hours, until pork is tender.

NUTRIENTS PER SERVING	
Calories	225
Fat	7.5 g
Saturates	2.2 g
Polyunsaturates	0.9 g
Monounsaturates	3.6 g
Cholesterol	53 mg
Sodium	483 mg
Carbohydrate	18.5 g
Fiber	5.3 g
Protein	20.8 g

AMERICA'S EXCHANGES	
1	Starch
2½	Lean Meat

CANADA'S CHOICES	
1	Carbohydrate
2½	Meat and Alternatives

Make Ahead

This dish can be partially prepared before it is cooked. Complete Steps 2 and 4, heating 1 tbsp (15 mL) oil in pan before softening the onions. Cover and refrigerate onion and chile mixtures separately for up to 2 days, being aware the chile mixture will lose some of its vibrancy if held for this long. (For best results, rehydrate chiles while the chili is cooking or no sooner than the night before you plan to cook.) When you're ready to cook, brown the pork, or if you're pressed for time, omit this step and continue with the recipe.

4. Half an hour before the recipe has finished cooking, in a heatproof bowl, soak ancho chiles in boiling water for 30 minutes, weighing down with a cup to ensure they remain submerged. Drain, discarding soaking liquid and stems, and chop coarsely. Transfer to a blender. Add cilantro, broth and chipotle pepper. Purée.

5. Add chile mixture to pork and stir well. Cover and cook on High for 30 minutes, until flavors meld. Ladle into bowls and garnish with sour cream and chopped onion, if using.

Mindful Morsels

Oregano, like many herbs, contains flavonoids, which act as antioxidants. Consumption of these antioxidants has been linked with reduced rates of heart disease and stroke. Although many culinary herbs act as antioxidants, USDA researchers have found oregano to have the most powerful antioxidant activity of the herbs they have studied.

Tip

To toast cumin seeds: Place seeds in a dry skillet over medium heat and cook, stirring, until fragrant and seeds just begin to brown, about 3 minutes. Immediately transfer to a mortar or a spice grinder and grind.

White Chicken Chili

Chili is one of my favorite weekday meals. I love its robust Tex-Mex flavors and the way the beans blend seamlessly with meat to create a sumptuous stew. This version, made from chicken and white beans, is lighter than traditional meat chilies. If you prefer a more colorful chili, use one red and one green bell pepper. Add a shredded carrot or sliced tomato salad, in season, and some whole grain bread to complete the meal.

- **Works best in a large (minimum 5 quart) slow cooker**

1 tbsp	olive oil	15 mL
2	onions, finely chopped	2
4	cloves garlic, minced	4
1 tbsp	cumin seeds, toasted and ground (see Tip, left)	15 mL
2 tsp	dried oregano leaves, crumbled	10 mL
1	piece (2 inches/5 cm) cinnamon stick	1
1 tsp	cracked black peppercorns	5 mL
2 cups	lower-salt chicken broth	500 mL
2 lbs	boneless skinless chicken thighs, quartered (about 12 thighs)	1 kg
2 cups	cooked dried or canned white kidney beans, drained and rinsed (see Basic Beans, page 231)	500 mL
2 tsp	dried ancho or New Mexico chile powder, dissolved in 1 tbsp (15 mL) freshly squeezed lime juice	10 mL
2	green bell peppers, finely chopped	2
1	jalapeño pepper, finely chopped	1
1	can (4½ oz/127 mL) diced mild green chiles, drained	1
1 cup	shredded light Monterey Jack cheese	250 mL
	Finely chopped cilantro	
	Lime wedges, optional	

1. In a skillet, heat oil over medium heat for 30 seconds. Add onions and cook, stirring, until softened, about 3 minutes. Add garlic, toasted cumin, oregano, cinnamon stick and peppercorns and cook, stirring, for 1 minute. Add broth and bring to a boil.

NUTRIENTS PER SERVING	
Calories	233
Fat	8.9 g
Saturates	3.1 g
Polyunsaturates	1.5 g
Monounsaturates	3.4 g
Cholesterol	69 mg
Sodium	372 mg
Carbohydrate	14.6 g
Fiber	5.0 g
Protein	23.7 g

AMERICA'S EXCHANGES	
1	Starch
3	Lean Meat

CANADA'S CHOICES	
½	Carbohydrate
3	Meat and Alternatives

Make Ahead

This dish can be partially prepared before it is cooked. Complete Step 1. Cover and refrigerate for up to 2 days. When you're ready to cook, continue with the recipe.

2. Transfer to slow cooker stoneware. Add chicken and beans and stir well. Cover and cook on Low for 6 hours or on High for 3 hours, until juices run clear when chicken is pierced with a fork.

3. Stir in chili powder solution. Add bell peppers, jalapeño pepper and green chiles and stir well. Cover and cook on High for 20 to 30 minutes, until peppers are tender. Add cheese and cook, stirring, until melted, about 1 minute. Ladle into bowls and garnish with cilantro. Pass lime wedges at the table, if using.

Mindful Morsels

Look for canned dried legumes, such as kidney beans, prepared without salt. If using regular beans, be sure to rinse them thoroughly and drain before use. When you have the time, prepare your own (see Basic Beans, page 231).

Tips

To toast cumin seeds: Place seeds in a dry skillet over medium heat and cook, stirring, until fragrant and seeds just begin to brown, about 3 minutes. Immediately transfer to a mortar or a spice grinder and grind.

Although they tend to be high in fat, used in small amounts, sausages are an easy way to add flavor to any dish.

Just about any chili powder works well in this recipe: ancho, New Mexico or a prepared blend.

Chorizo is usually quite spicy, so add the jalapeño only if you're a heat seeker.

Chicken Chili and Barley Casserole

This flavorful dish, which bridges the gap between chicken chili and a baked casserole, is a hit with all family members. It's a great dish for those evenings when everyone is coming and going at different times. Just leave the slow cooker setting on Warm and the fixings for salad.

- **Large (minimum 5 quart) slow cooker**

1 tbsp	olive oil	15 mL
2	fresh chorizo sausages, casings removed and crumbled (about 4 oz/125 g total)	2
2	onions, finely chopped	2
4	cloves garlic, minced	4
1 tsp	dried oregano leaves, crumbled	5 mL
1 tsp	cracked black peppercorns	5 mL
1 tbsp	cumin seeds, toasted and ground (see Tips, left)	15 mL
1	can (28 oz/796 mL) diced tomatoes, including juice	1
2 cups	lower-salt chicken broth	500 mL
1 cup	whole (hulled) or pot barley, rinsed	250 mL
1	can (14 oz/398 mL) white beans, drained and rinsed	1
1 lb	boneless skinless chicken thighs, cut into bite-size pieces	500 g
2	red bell peppers, diced	2
2 tsp	chili powder, dissolved in 1 tbsp (15 mL) lime juice (see Tips, left)	10 mL
1	jalapeño pepper, seeded and minced, optional (see Tips, left)	1
1 cup	diced avocado (about 1)	250 mL
2 tbsp	freshly squeezed lime juice	25 mL
	Finely chopped red onion and cilantro	

1. In a large skillet, heat oil over medium heat for 30 seconds. Add sausage and onions and cook, stirring, until onions are softened and no hint of pink remains in sausage, about 4 minutes. Add garlic, oregano, peppercorns and toasted cumin and cook, stirring, for 1 minute. Add tomatoes with juice and bring to a boil. Transfer to slow cooker stoneware.

NUTRIENTS PER SERVING	
Calories	244
Fat	9.4 g
Saturates	2.5 g
Polyunsaturates	1.4 g
Monounsaturates	4.6 g
Cholesterol	34 mg
Sodium	426 mg
Carbohydrate	27.5 g
Fiber	5.0 g
Protein	14.0 g

AMERICA'S EXCHANGES	
2	Starch
1½	Lean Meat
½	Fat

CANADA'S CHOICES	
1½	Carbohydrate
1½	Meat and Alternatives
1	Fat

Make Ahead

This dish can be partially prepared before it is cooked. Complete Step 1. Cover and refrigerate overnight or for up to 2 days. When you're ready to cook, continue with Steps 2 and 3.

2. Add broth, barley, beans and chicken and stir well. Cover and cook on Low for 6 hours or on High for 3 hours, until juices run clear when chicken is pierced with a fork and barley is tender. Stir in bell peppers, chili powder solution and jalapeño pepper, if using. Cover and cook for 20 minutes, until peppers are tender.

3. Meanwhile, in a bowl, combine avocado and lime juice. To serve, ladle casserole onto plates, top with avocado mixture and garnish with onion and cilantro.

Mindful Morsels

Avocados are high in fat, but only a small amount of it is saturated. They also contain significant amounts of other nutrients. Half a Haas avocado is low in sodium, is an excellent source of folacin, and is high in fiber, vitamin E, pantothenic acid, vitamin K and potassium.

Tips

You can also make this chili using leftover turkey. Use 3 cups (750 mL) of shredded cooked turkey and add along with the bell peppers.

To toast cumin seeds: Place seeds in a dry skillet over medium heat and cook, stirring, until fragrant and seeds just begin to brown, about 3 minutes. Immediately transfer to a mortar or a spice grinder and grind.

Make Ahead

This dish can be partially prepared before it is cooked. Complete Step 1. Cover and refrigerate overnight or for up to 2 days. When you're ready to cook, continue with Steps 2 and 3.

Two-Bean Turkey Chili

This delicious chili, which has just a hint of heat, is perfect for family get-togethers. Add a tossed green salad, sprinkled with shredded carrots, and whole grain rolls.

- **Works in slow cookers from 3½ to 6 quarts**

1 tbsp	olive oil	15 mL
2	onions, finely chopped	2
4	stalks celery, diced	4
6	cloves garlic, minced	6
2 tsp	dried oregano leaves, crumbled	10 mL
½ tsp	cracked black peppercorns	2 mL
	Zest of 1 lime	
1 tbsp	cumin seeds, toasted and ground (see Tips, left)	15 mL
2 tbsp	fine cornmeal	25 mL
1 cup	lower-salt chicken broth	250 mL
1	can (28 oz/796 mL) diced tomatoes, including juice	1
2 lbs	bone-in turkey breast, skin removed, cut into ½-inch (1 cm) cubes (about 3 cups/750 mL)	1 kg
2	cans (each 14 oz/398 mL) pinto beans, drained and rinsed	2
2 cups	frozen sliced green beans	500 mL
1 tbsp	New Mexico or ancho chili powder, dissolved in 2 tbsp (25 mL) lime juice	15 mL
1	each green and red bell pepper, diced	1
1	can (4½ oz/127 mL) diced mild green chiles	1

1. In a skillet, heat oil over medium heat for 30 seconds. Add onions and celery and cook, stirring, until celery is softened, about 5 minutes. Add garlic and cook, stirring, for 1 minute. Add oregano, peppercorns, lime zest and toasted cumin and cook, stirring, for 1 minute. Add cornmeal and toss to coat. Add broth and cook, stirring, until mixture boils, about 1 minute. Add tomatoes with juice and return to a boil. Transfer to slow cooker stoneware.

2. Add turkey, pinto beans and green beans and stir well. Cover and cook on Low for 8 hours or on High for 4 hours, until turkey is tender and mixture is bubbly.

3. Add chili powder solution, green and red bell peppers and mild green chiles. Cover and cook on High for 30 minutes, until bell peppers are tender.

NUTRIENTS PER SERVING	
Calories	238
Fat	4.1 g
Saturates	1.0 g
Polyunsaturates	0.8 g
Monounsaturates	1.9 g
Cholesterol	37 mg
Sodium	547 mg
Carbohydrate	28.1 g
Fiber	7.7 g
Protein	23.5 g

AMERICA'S EXCHANGES	
1	Starch
2	Vegetable
2½	Very Lean Meat

CANADA'S CHOICES	
1	Carbohydrate
2½	Meat and Alternatives

Vegetarian Main Courses

**MAKES ABOUT
8 CUPS (2 L)**
(1 cup/250 mL per serving)

Tip

If you are in a hurry, you can soften the vegetables on the stovetop. Heat oil in a skillet for 30 seconds. Add onions and carrots and cook, stirring, until carrots are softened, about 7 minutes. Add garlic, thyme and peppercorns and cook, stirring, for 1 minute. Transfer to slow cooker stoneware. Add tomatoes with juice and continue with Step 2.

Basic Tomato Sauce

Not only is this sauce tasty and easy to make, it is also much lower in sodium than prepared sauces. It keeps covered for up to 1 week in the refrigerator and can be frozen for up to 6 months.

- **Works in slow cookers from 3½ to 6 quarts**

1 tbsp	olive oil	15 mL
2	onions, finely chopped	2
2	carrots, peeled and diced	2
4	cloves garlic, minced	4
1 tsp	dried thyme leaves, crumbled	5 mL
½ tsp	cracked black peppercorns	2 mL
2	cans (each 28 oz/796 mL) diced tomatoes, including juice	2

1. In slow cooker stoneware, combine olive oil, onions and carrots. Stir well to ensure vegetables are coated with oil. Cover and cook on High for 1 hour, until vegetables are softened. Add garlic, thyme and peppercorns. Stir well. Stir in tomatoes with juice.

2. Place a tea towel folded in half (so you have two layers) over top of stoneware to absorb moisture. Cover and cook on Low for 6 to 8 hours or on High for 3 to 4 hours, until sauce is thickened and flavors are melded.

Mindful Morsels

One advantage to making your own tomato sauce is that it is much lower in sodium than prepared versions. One-half cup (125 mL) of prepared tomato sauce, a typical serving size when used in a recipe, may contain as much as 700 mg of sodium. One-half cup (125 mL) of this sauce with no added salt contains approximately 155 mg of sodium. If you want to reduce your intake of sodium even further, make this sauce using canned tomatoes with no salt added, which are now widely available.

NUTRIENTS PER SERVING	
Calories	75
Fat	2.1 g
Saturates	0.3 g
Polyunsaturates	0.3 g
Monounsaturates	1.3 g
Cholesterol	0 mg
Sodium	311 mg
Carbohydrate	13.8 g
Fiber	2.6 g
Protein	2.5 g

AMERICA'S EXCHANGES	
1	Vegetable
½	Other Carbohydrate
½	Fat

CANADA'S CHOICES	
1	Carbohydrate
½	Fat

Mushroom Tomato Sauce

MAKES 6 SERVINGS

Tip

For an easy and delicious meal, make this sauce ahead of time and refrigerate. Prepare 1 batch of Basic Polenta (see page 229), and just before it is ready to serve, reheat Mushroom Tomato Sauce. To serve, spoon polenta onto a warm plate and top with the sauce.

Make Ahead

This dish can be partially prepared before it is cooked. Complete Step 1. Cover and refrigerate overnight or for up to 2 days. When you're ready to cook, continue with Step 2.

One way of adding variety to your diet is by expanding the kinds of grains you use with sauces traditionally served with pasta. I like to serve this classic sauce over polenta (see page 229) or whole wheat pasta. Accompanied by a tossed green salad, it makes a great weeknight meal.

- **Works in slow cookers from 3½ to 6 quarts**

1 tbsp	olive oil	15 mL
1	onion, finely chopped	1
2	stalks celery, diced	2
4	cloves garlic, minced	4
1 tbsp	finely chopped fresh rosemary or 2 tsp (10 mL) dried rosemary leaves, crumbled	15 mL
½ tsp	salt	2 mL
½ tsp	cracked black peppercorns	2 mL
8 oz	cremini mushrooms, sliced	250 g
½ cup	dry white wine or lower-salt chicken or vegetable broth	125 mL
1 tbsp	tomato paste	15 mL
1	can (28 oz/796 mL) diced tomatoes, including juice	1
	Crushed red pepper flakes, optional	
	Freshly grated Parmesan cheese, optional	

1. In a skillet, heat oil over medium heat for 30 seconds. Add onion and celery and cook, stirring, until celery is softened, about 5 minutes. Add garlic, rosemary, salt and peppercorns and cook, stirring, for 1 minute. Add mushrooms and toss to coat. Add wine and cook for 1 minute. Stir in tomato paste and tomatoes with juice and bring to a boil. Transfer to slow cooker stoneware.

2. Place a tea towel folded in half (so you will have two layers) over top of the stoneware to absorb moisture. Cover and cook on Low for 6 hours or on High for 3 hours, until hot and bubbly. Stir in pepper flakes, if using. Serve over cooked whole wheat pasta, polenta or grits. Garnish with Parmesan to taste, if using.

NUTRIENTS PER SERVING	
Calories	67
Fat	2.6 g
Saturates	0.4 g
Polyunsaturates	0.3 g
Monounsaturates	1.7 g
Cholesterol	0 mg
Sodium	403 mg
Carbohydrate	10.5 g
Fiber	2.3 g
Protein	2.5 g

AMERICA'S EXCHANGES	
2	Vegetable
½	Fat

CANADA'S CHOICES	
½	Fat

Celery Root and Mushroom Lasagna

Tip

Make this using whole wheat lasagna noodles or oven-ready noodles, if you prefer. If using oven-ready noodles, do not toss with olive oil and use only 1 tbsp (15 mL) of oil when softening the vegetables.

If you're tired of the same old thing, try this delightfully different lasagna, which combines celery root and mushrooms with more traditional tomatoes and cheese.

- **Large (minimum 5 quart) oval slow cooker**
- **Greased slow cooker stoneware**

9	brown rice lasagna noodles (see Tip, left)	9
2 tbsp	extra virgin olive oil, divided	25 mL
4 cups	shredded peeled celery root (about 1 medium celery root)	1 L
2 tbsp	freshly squeezed lemon juice	25 mL
1	large sweet onion, such as Spanish or Vidalia, finely chopped	1
1 lb	cremini mushrooms, stems removed and caps sliced	500 g
4	cloves garlic, minced	4
1 tbsp	fresh thyme leaves or 1 tsp (5 mL) dried thyme leaves, crumbled	15 mL
1 tbsp	fresh rosemary leaves, finely chopped, or 1 tsp (5 mL) dried rosemary leaves, crumbled	15 mL
4 cups	Basic Tomato Sauce (see recipe, page 106), divided	1 L
1	container (16 oz/475 g) light (5%) ricotta cheese	1
2 cups	shredded part-skim mozzarella cheese	500 mL

1. Cook lasagna noodles in a pot of boiling salted water until slightly undercooked, or according to package instructions, undercooking by 2 minutes. Drain, toss with 1 tbsp (15 mL) of the oil and set aside.

2. In a bowl, toss celery root with lemon juice. Set aside.

3. In a skillet, heat remaining 1 tbsp (15 mL) of the oil over medium heat for 30 seconds. Add onion and mushrooms and cook, stirring, for 2 minutes. Add garlic, thyme and rosemary and cook, stirring, for 1 minute. Add celery root and 2 cups (500 mL) of the tomato sauce and bring to a boil. Remove from heat.

NUTRIENTS PER SERVING	
Calories	287
Fat	11.6 g
Saturates	5.2 g
Polyunsaturates	0.9 g
Monounsaturates	4.8 g
Cholesterol	23 mg
Sodium	348 mg
Carbohydrate	30.4 g
Fiber	4.1 g
Protein	16.4 g

AMERICA'S EXCHANGES	
1	Starch
3	Vegetable
1½	Medium-fat Meat
1	Fat

CANADA'S CHOICES	
2	Carbohydrate
1½	Meat and Alternatives
1½	Fat

Make Ahead

This dish can be partially prepared before it is cooked. Complete Steps 1 through 4. Cover and refrigerate overnight. In the morning, continue with Step 5.

4. Spread 1 cup (250 mL) of the tomato sauce over bottom of prepared slow cooker stoneware. Cover with 3 noodles. Spread with half of the ricotta, half of the mushroom mixture and one-third of the mozzarella. Repeat. Cover with final layer of noodles. Pour remaining 1 cup (250 mL) of the tomato sauce over top. Sprinkle with remaining mozzarella.

5. Cover and cook on Low for 6 hours or on High for 3 hours, until mushrooms are tender and mixture is hot and bubbly.

MAKES 8 SERVINGS

Tips

Celery root oxidizes quickly on contact with air. Tossing it with lemon juice keeps it from discoloring.

To clean leeks: Fill a sink full of lukewarm water. Split the leeks in half lengthwise and submerge them in the water, swishing them around to remove all traces of dirt. Transfer to a colander and rinse thoroughly under cold water.

If your supermarket carries 19-oz (540 mL) cans of diced tomatoes, by all means substitute for the 14-oz (398 mL) can called for in the recipe.

Although pearl barley is more readily available, make an effort to find whole (also known as hulled) barley when making the recipes in this book. It contains more nutrients, including fiber, than its refined relative. Pot barley, which is more refined than whole barley, is also a preferable alternative to pearl barley as it maintains some of the bran.

Winter Vegetable Casserole

Here's a great dish to make during the dark days of winter. The combination of root vegetables, seasoned with caraway seeds, produces a great-tasting dish that is seasonally appropriate — I like to imagine my pioneer ancestors sitting down to a similar meal. I serve this with rye bread and steamed broccoli.

- **Large (minimum 5 quart) slow cooker**

1	large celery root, peeled and shredded	1
1 tbsp	freshly squeezed lemon juice	15 mL
1 tbsp	olive oil	15 mL
2	leeks, white and light green parts only, cleaned and thinly sliced (see Tips, left)	2
4	carrots, peeled and sliced	4
4	parsnips, peeled and sliced	4
2	cloves garlic, minced	2
1 tsp	caraway seeds	5 mL
1 tsp	salt	5 mL
½ tsp	cracked black peppercorns	2 mL
1	can (14 oz/398 mL) diced tomatoes, including juice (see Tips, left)	1
2 cups	lower-salt vegetable broth	500 mL
½ cup	whole (hulled) or pot barley (see Tips, left)	125 mL
½ cup	finely chopped parsley leaves	125 mL

1. In a bowl, toss celery root and lemon juice. Set aside.

2. In a large skillet, heat oil over medium heat for 30 seconds. Add leeks, carrots and parsnips and cook, stirring, until vegetables have softened, about 7 minutes. Add garlic, caraway seeds, salt and peppercorns and cook, stirring, for 1 minute. Add tomatoes with juice, broth and barley and bring to a boil.

3. Spread celery root over bottom of slow cooker. Add vegetable mixture and stir well. Cover and cook on Low for 6 hours or on High for 3 hours, until vegetables and barley are tender. Sprinkle with parsley and serve.

NUTRIENTS PER SERVING

Calories	173
Fat	2.6 g
Saturates	0.4 g
Polyunsaturates	0.5 g
Monounsaturates	1.4 g
Cholesterol	0 mg
Sodium	438 mg
Carbohydrate	35.9 g
Fiber	6.3 g
Protein	4.0 g

AMERICA'S EXCHANGES	
1	Starch
4	Vegetable

CANADA'S CHOICES	
2	Carbohydrate
½	Fat

Vegetable Stroganoff

This robust stew makes a delicious dinner with a salad and crusty bread. You can also serve it over hot whole wheat fettuccine or brown rice noodles.

MAKES 8 SERVINGS

Tips

If you're using portobello mushrooms, discard the stem, cut the caps into quarters and thinly slice. If you're using cremini mushrooms, trim off the tough end of the stem and cut them into quarters. Save the stems for making vegetable stock.

Use only good-quality blue cheese such as Maytag or Italian Gorgonzola for this recipe as blue cheese of lesser quality tends to be very harsh.

If you are in a hurry, warm the cream and cheese before adding to the stoneware. Stir in and serve as soon as the cheese melts.

Make Ahead

This dish can be partially prepared before it is cooked. Complete Step 1. Cover and refrigerate for up to 2 days. When you're ready to cook, continue with the recipe.

- **Works best in a large (minimum 5 quart) slow cooker**

1 tbsp	olive oil	15 mL
2	large leeks, white part only, cleaned and thinly sliced (see Tips, page 110)	2
4	stalks celery, thinly sliced	4
2	cloves garlic, minced	2
1 tsp	dried thyme leaves	5 mL
1 tsp	cracked black peppercorns	5 mL
½ tsp	salt	2 mL
1	can (28 oz/796 mL) diced tomatoes, including juice	1
1 cup	lower-salt vegetable broth	250 mL
1 lb	portobello or cremini mushrooms, stems removed and caps sliced (see Tips, left)	500 g
2	potatoes, peeled and cut into ½-inch (1 cm) cubes	2
¼ cup	whipping (35%) cream	50 mL
2 oz	good-quality blue cheese, crumbled, and at room temperature (see Tips, left)	60 g

1. In a skillet, heat oil over medium heat. Add leeks and celery and cook, stirring, until softened, about 5 minutes. Add garlic, thyme, peppercorns and salt and cook, stirring, for 1 minute. Add tomatoes, with juice, and broth and bring to a boil. Transfer to slow cooker stoneware.

2. Stir in mushrooms and potatoes. Cover and cook on Low for 8 to 10 hours or on High for 4 to 5 hours, until potatoes are tender. Stir in cream and cheese. Cover and cook on High for 15 minutes, or until cheese is melted into sauce and mixture is hot and bubbly.

NUTRIENTS PER SERVING	
Calories	142
Fat	7.0 g
Saturates	3.3 g
Polyunsaturates	0.6 g
Monounsaturates	2.6 g
Cholesterol	15 mg
Sodium	494 mg
Carbohydrate	17.6 g
Fiber	3.9 g
Protein	4.8 g

AMERICA'S EXCHANGES	
½	Starch
2	Vegetable
1½	Fat

CANADA'S CHOICES	
1	Carbohydrate
1½	Fat

Vegetable Goulash

MAKES 6 SERVINGS

Make Ahead

This dish can be partially prepared before it is cooked. Complete Steps 1, 2 and 3. Cover and refrigerate for up to 2 days. When you're ready to cook, continue with the recipe.

Variation

Vegetable Pot Pie: If desired, add ½ cup (125 mL) whipping (35%) cream to the cooked goulash. Ladle into a casserole dish or 4 ovenproof ramekins. Top with thawed prepared puff pastry, cut to fit. Bake for 20 to 25 minutes in a 400°F (200°C) oven, until pastry is puffed and browned.

This hearty and delicious stew is the perfect pick-me-up after a day in the chilly outdoors. Serve over hot whole wheat fettuccine or brown rice noodles, topped with a dollop of sour cream, if desired. Accompany with dark rye bread and a salad of shredded carrots. For a special occasion, see Variation, left.

• Works in slow cookers from 3½ to 6 quarts

4	dried shiitake mushrooms	4
1 cup	hot water	250 mL
2 tbsp	olive oil, divided	25 mL
8 oz	fresh shiitake mushrooms, stems removed and caps coarsely chopped	250 g
1	onion, finely chopped	1
4	stalks celery, diced	4
2	carrots, peeled and diced	2
2	parsnips, peeled and diced	2
1 tsp	caraway seeds, coarsely crushed	5 mL
½ tsp	salt	2 mL
½ tsp	cracked black peppercorns	2 mL
1 tbsp	all-purpose flour	15 mL
2 cups	lower-salt vegetable broth	500 mL
2 tsp	paprika	10 mL
1	green bell pepper, seeded and diced	1

1. Soak dried mushrooms in hot water for 30 minutes. Drain and pat dry. Cut into quarters.

2. In a skillet, heat 1 tbsp (15 mL) of the oil over medium heat for 30 seconds. Add fresh mushrooms and cook, stirring, for 1 minute. Transfer to slow cooker stoneware.

3. Heat remaining oil in pan. Add onion, celery, carrots and parsnips and cook, stirring, until softened, about 7 minutes. Add caraway seeds, salt, peppercorns and reserved dried shiitake mushrooms and cook, stirring, for 1 minute. Add flour and cook, stirring, for 1 minute. Add broth and cook, stirring, until thickened, about 3 minutes. Transfer to slow cooker stoneware.

4. Cover and cook on Low for 6 hours or on High for 3 hours, until vegetables are tender. Stir in paprika and green pepper. Cover and cook on High until pepper is soft, about 15 minutes.

NUTRIENTS PER SERVING	
Calories	134
Fat	5.2 g
Saturates	0.7 g
Polyunsaturates	0.6 g
Monounsaturates	3.4 g
Cholesterol	0 mg
Sodium	388 mg
Carbohydrate	21.7 g
Fiber	3.9 g
Protein	2.6 g

AMERICA'S EXCHANGES	
4	Vegetable
1	Fat

CANADA'S CHOICES	
1	Carbohydrate
1	Fat

MAKES 10 SERVINGS

Tips

To toast cumin and coriander seeds: Place seeds in a dry skillet over medium heat and toast, stirring, until fragrant and cumin seeds just begin to brown, about 3 minutes. Immediately transfer to a mortar or a spice grinder and grind.

If using fresh spinach, be sure to remove the stems, and if it has not been pre-washed, rinse it thoroughly in a basin of lukewarm water.

Make Ahead

This dish can be partially prepared before it is cooked. Complete Step 1. Cover and refrigerate overnight or for up to 2 days. When you're ready to cook, continue with Step 2.

NUTRIENTS PER SERVING	
Calories	194
Fat	2.6 g
Saturates	0.4 g
Polyunsaturates	0.6 g
Monounsaturates	1.3 g
Cholesterol	0 mg
Sodium	368 mg
Carbohydrate	35.1 g
Fiber	6.2 g
Protein	9.3 g

Spinach Dal with Millet

Dal, which is usually made with split yellow peas, is one of my favorite ethnic comfort foods. Usually served as one of several small dishes at an Indian meal, dal is very versatile. I often enjoy it as a main course, accompanied by a tossed salad. It also makes a delicious side to accompany grilled or roasted chicken or meat.

- **Large (minimum 5 quart) slow cooker**

1 tbsp	olive oil	15 mL
2	onions, finely chopped	2
4	cloves garlic, minced	4
1 tbsp	minced gingerroot	15 mL
1 tsp	turmeric	5 mL
1/2 tsp	cracked black peppercorns	2 mL
2	bay leaves	2
1 tbsp	cumin seeds, toasted (see Tips, left)	15 mL
2 tsp	coriander seeds, toasted	10 mL
1	can (28 oz/796 mL) diced tomatoes, including juice	1
3 cups	lower-salt vegetable broth	750 mL
1 cup	red lentils, rinsed	250 mL
1 cup	millet, rinsed	250 mL
1/4 tsp	cayenne, dissolved in 2 tbsp (25 mL) freshly squeezed lemon juice	1 mL
1 lb	fresh spinach, stems removed, or 1 package (10 oz/300 g) fresh or frozen spinach, thawed and drained if frozen (see Tips, left)	500 g
	Low-fat plain yogurt, optional	
1/4 cup	finely chopped cilantro leaves	50 mL

1. In a skillet, heat oil over medium heat. Add onions and cook, stirring, until softened, about 3 minutes. Add garlic and gingerroot and cook, stirring, for 1 minute. Add turmeric, peppercorns, bay leaves and toasted cumin and coriander and cook, stirring, for 1 minute. Add tomatoes with juice and bring to a boil. Transfer to slow cooker stoneware.

2. Add broth, lentils and millet and stir well. Cover and cook on Low for 10 hours or on High for 5 hours, until lentils are tender. Stir in cayenne solution. Add spinach, in batches, stirring after each batch, until all the leaves are submerged in the liquid. Cover and cook on High for 20 minutes, until spinach is tender. Discard bay leaves. Transfer to a large serving bowl, drizzle with yogurt, if using, and garnish with cilantro.

AMERICA'S EXCHANGES	
2	Starch
1	Vegetable
1/2	Lean Meat

CANADA'S CHOICES	
2	Carbohydrate
1/2	Meat and Alternatives

MAKES 8 SERVINGS

MAKES 8 SERVINGS

Tip

If using fresh spinach, be sure to remove the stems, and if it has not been pre-washed, rinse it thoroughly in a basin of lukewarm water.

Vegetable Curry with Lentils and Spinach

Serve this delicious curry for dinner with warm Indian bread such as naan. It's a meal in itself.

- **Large (minimum 5 quart) slow cooker**

2 tsp	cumin seeds	10 mL
1 tsp	coriander seeds	5 mL
1 tbsp	olive oil or extra virgin coconut oil	15 mL
2	onions, finely chopped	2
4	carrots, peeled and thinly sliced (about 1 lb/500 g)	4
4	parsnips, peeled and tough core removed, thinly sliced (about 1 lb/500 g)	4
4	cloves garlic, minced	4
1 tbsp	minced gingerroot	15 mL
2 tsp	turmeric	10 mL
1	piece (2 inches/5 cm) cinnamon stick	1
½ tsp	cracked black peppercorns	2 mL
2 cups	lower-salt vegetable broth	500 mL
2	sweet potatoes, peeled and thinly sliced (about 1 lb/500 g)	2
1 cup	brown or green lentils, picked over and rinsed	250 mL
1	long red chile pepper, finely chopped, or ½ tsp (2 mL) cayenne pepper, dissolved in 1 tbsp (15 mL) lemon juice	1
1 lb	fresh spinach, stems removed, or 1 package (10 oz/300 g) spinach leaves, thawed and drained if frozen, coarsely chopped (see Tip, left)	500 g
1 cup	coconut milk, optional (see Mindful Morsels, right)	250 mL

1. In a dry skillet over medium heat, toast cumin and coriander seeds until fragrant and cumin seeds just begin to brown, about 3 minutes. Immediately transfer to a mortar or a spice grinder and grind. Set aside.

2. In same skillet, heat oil over medium heat for 30 seconds. Add onions, carrots and parsnips and cook, stirring, until vegetables are tender, about 6 minutes. Add garlic, gingerroot, turmeric, cinnamon stick, peppercorns and reserved cumin and coriander and cook, stirring, for 1 minute. Add broth and bring to a boil. Transfer to slow cooker stoneware. Add sweet potatoes and lentils and stir well.

NUTRIENTS PER SERVING	
Calories	252
Fat	2.7 g
Saturates	0.4 g
Polyunsaturates	0.5 g
Monounsaturates	1.5 g
Cholesterol	0 mg
Sodium	253 mg
Carbohydrate	49.6 g
Fiber	8.7 g
Protein	10 g

AMERICA'S EXCHANGES	
2½	Starch
2	Vegetable

CANADA'S CHOICES	
2½	Carbohydrate
½	Meat and Alternatives

Make Ahead

This dish can be partially prepared before it is cooked. Complete Steps 1 and 2. Cover and refrigerate overnight or for up to 2 days. When you're ready to cook, continue with Step 3.

3. Cover and cook on Low for 8 hours or on High for 4 hours, until lentils are tender. Add chile pepper and stir well. Add spinach, in batches, stirring after each batch until all the leaves are submerged in the liquid, then coconut milk, if using. Cover and cook on High for 20 minutes, until spinach is wilted and flavors have blended. Discard cinnamon stick.

Mindful Morsels

The coconut milk adds a pleasant nutty flavor and creaminess to the curry, but it is high in saturated fat. The curry is very tasty on its own, so you can omit the coconut milk if you prefer.

Vegetable Cobbler with Millet Crust

Not only is this tasty cobbler loaded with flavor, the distinctive millet crust adds whole grain goodness to this delightfully different treat. Add a sliced tomato salad, in season, or a tossed green salad topped with shredded carrots to add color and nutrients.

Tips

Like lentils, some millet may contain bits of dirt or discolored grains. If your millet looks grimy, rinse it thoroughly in a pot of water before using. Swish it around and remove any offending particles, then rinse under cold running water.

You can substitute 1 tbsp (15 mL) dried rosemary leaves, crumbled, for the fresh.

If using canned beans in this recipe, be sure to rinse them thoroughly under cold running water to remove as much sodium as possible.

Variation

Although it makes this dish unsuitable for vegetarians, I find that adding a small bit of pancetta (Italian-style cured pork) adds a tremendous amount of flavor. I use a 3-oz (90 g) chunk, diced and sautéed in the olive oil until it becomes crispy, about 3 minutes. Then I add the onions, carrots and celery.

* **Large (minimum 6 quart) slow cooker**

Topping

1 cup	millet (see Tips, left)	250 mL
3 cups	water	750 mL
	Freshly ground black pepper	
½ cup	freshly grated Parmesan, optional	125 mL

Cobbler

1 tbsp	olive oil	15 mL
2	onions, finely chopped	2
4	carrots, peeled and diced	4
4	stalks celery, diced	4
2 tbsp	fresh rosemary leaves, finely chopped	25 mL
4	cloves garlic, minced	4
½ tsp	cracked black peppercorns	2 mL
1	can (28 oz/796 mL) diced tomatoes, including juice	1
1	can (14 to 19 oz/398 to 540 mL) white beans, drained and rinsed (see Tips, left), or 1 cup (250 mL) dried white beans, soaked, cooked and drained (see Basic Beans, page 231)	1
12 oz	frozen sliced green beans (about 2 cups/ 500 mL)	375 g

1. **Topping:** In a saucepan over medium heat, toast millet, stirring constantly, until it crackles and releases its aroma, about 5 minutes. Add water, and black pepper to taste, and bring to a boil. Reduce heat to low, cover and cook until millet is tender and all the water is absorbed, about 20 minutes. Stir in Parmesan, if using, and set aside.

NUTRIENTS PER SERVING	
Calories	220
Fat	3.2 g
Saturates	0.5 g
Polyunsaturates	0.8 g
Monounsaturates	1.5 g
Cholesterol	0 mg
Sodium	335 mg
Carbohydrate	42.0 g
Fiber	8.4 g
Protein	8.4 g

AMERICA'S EXCHANGES	
2	Starch
2	Vegetable
½	Fat

CANADA'S CHOICES	
2	Carbohydrate
1	Fat

Make Ahead

This dish can be partially prepared before it is cooked. Complete Step 2. Cover and refrigerate overnight or for up to 2 days. When you're ready to cook, continue with Steps 1 and 3.

2. **Cobbler:** Meanwhile, in a large skillet, heat oil over medium heat for 30 seconds. Add onions, carrots and celery and cook, stirring, until vegetables are softened, about 7 minutes. Add rosemary, garlic and peppercorns and cook, stirring, for 1 minute. Add tomatoes with juice and bring to a boil. Transfer to stoneware.

3. Add white beans and green beans and stir well. Spread millet evenly over the top. Cover and cook on Low for 8 to 10 hours or on High for 4 to 5 hours, until hot and bubbly.

MAKES 6 SERVINGS

Tips

Large cans of tomatoes come in 28 oz (796 mL) and 35 oz (980 mL) sizes. For convenience, I've called for the 28 oz (796 mL) size in my recipes. If you're using the 35 oz (980 mL) size, drain off 1 cup (250 mL) liquid before adding to the recipe.

For convenience, use bottled roasted red peppers, or, if you prefer, roast your own.

Mushroom and Chickpea Stew with Roasted Red Pepper Coulis

I've served this delicious stew to nonvegetarians who have scraped the bowl. Topped with the luscious coulis, it is quite divine. Add whole grain rolls and a green salad or steamed asparagus, in season.

- **Works in slow cookers from 3½ to 6 quarts**

1 tbsp	cumin seeds	15 mL
1 tbsp	olive oil	15 mL
2	onions, finely chopped	2
2	carrots, peeled and diced	2
4	stalks celery, thinly sliced, or 1 bulb fennel, trimmed, cored and thinly sliced on the vertical	4
4	cloves garlic, minced	4
1 tsp	turmeric	5 mL
¼ tsp	salt	1 mL
½ tsp	cracked black peppercorns	2 mL
8 oz	cremini mushrooms, thinly sliced	250 g
1	can (28 oz/796 mL) diced tomatoes, including juice (see Tips, left)	1
1	can (14 oz/398 mL) chickpeas, drained and rinsed, or 1 cup (250 mL) dried chickpeas, soaked, cooked and drained (see Variation, page 231)	1

Red Pepper Coulis

2	roasted red bell peppers (see Tips, left)	2
3	oil-packed sun-dried tomatoes, drained and chopped	3
2 tbsp	extra virgin olive oil	25 mL
1 tbsp	balsamic vinegar	15 mL
10	fresh basil leaves, optional	10

1. In a large dry skillet over medium heat, toast cumin seeds, stirring, until fragrant and they just begin to brown, about 3 minutes. Immediately transfer to a mortar or a spice grinder and grind. Set aside.

NUTRIENTS PER SERVING	
Calories	202
Fat	7.5 g
Saturates	1.0 g
Polyunsaturates	1.0 g
Monounsaturates	4.9 g
Cholesterol	0 mg
Sodium	558 mg
Carbohydrate	30.5 g
Fiber	6.5 g
Protein	6.5 g

AMERICA'S EXCHANGES	
1½	Starch
2	Vegetable
1	Fat

CANADA'S CHOICES	
1½	Carbohydrate
½	Meat and Alternatives
1	Fat

Make Ahead

This dish can be partially prepared before it is cooked. Complete Steps 1 and 2. Cover and refrigerate overnight or for up to 2 days. When you're ready to cook, continue with Steps 3 and 4.

2. In same skillet, heat oil over medium heat for 30 seconds. Add onions, carrots and celery and cook, stirring, until vegetables are tender, about 7 minutes. Add garlic, turmeric, salt, peppercorns and reserved cumin and cook, stirring, for 1 minute. Add mushrooms and toss until coated. Add tomatoes with juice and bring to a boil. Transfer to slow cooker stoneware.

3. Add chickpeas and stir well. Cover and cook on Low for 6 hours or on High for 3 hours, until hot and bubbly.

4. Roasted Red Pepper Coulis: In a food processor, combine roasted peppers, sun-dried tomatoes, oil, vinegar, and basil, if using. Process until smooth. Ladle stew into bowls and top with coulis.

Mindful Morsels

Most of the sodium in a serving of this recipe comes from the canned tomatoes (200 mg), the canned chickpeas (135 mg) and, of course, the salt (100 mg). There are several ways you can reduce the amount of sodium from these ingredients in any recipe: use tomatoes and/or chickpeas canned without salt; use fresh tomatoes in season; prepare homemade stock from scratch without salt; and cut back on added salt.

MAKES 6 SERVINGS

Tips

I prefer a strong gingery flavor in this dish. If you're ginger-averse, reduce the amount.

Large cans of tomatoes come in 28 oz (796 mL) and 35 oz (980 mL) sizes. For convenience, I've called for the 28 oz (796 mL) size in my recipes. If you're using the 35 oz (980 mL) size, drain off 1 cup (250 mL) liquid before adding to the recipe.

Tagine of Squash and Chickpeas with Mushrooms

I love the unusual combination of flavorings in this dish, which meld beautifully. The taste of the cinnamon and ginger really come through, and the bittersweet combination of lemon and honey adds a perfect finish. Serve this over whole grain couscous to complete the Middle Eastern flavors and provide vegetarians with a complete protein. Add a leafy green vegetable, such as spinach or Swiss chard, to complete the meal.

* **Works in slow cookers from 3½ to 6 quarts**

1 tbsp	olive oil	15 mL
1	onion, finely chopped	1
2	carrots, peeled and diced (about 1 cup/250 mL)	2
4	cloves garlic, minced	4
2 tbsp	minced gingerroot (see Tips, left)	25 mL
1 tsp	turmeric	5 mL
½ tsp	salt	2 mL
½ tsp	cracked black peppercorns	2 mL
1	piece (2 inches/5 cm) cinnamon stick	1
8 oz	cremini mushrooms, stemmed and halved	250 g
1	can (28 oz/796 mL) diced tomatoes, including juice (see Tips, left)	1
3 cups	cubed (1 inch/2.5 cm) peeled butternut squash or pumpkin	750 mL
2 cups	cooked dried chickpeas (see Variation, page 231) or canned chickpeas, drained and rinsed	500 mL
1 tbsp	liquid honey	15 mL
1 tbsp	freshly squeezed lemon juice	15 mL

1. In a large skillet, heat oil over medium heat for 30 seconds. Add onion and carrots and cook, stirring, until carrots are softened, about 7 minutes. Add garlic, gingerroot, turmeric, salt, peppercorns and cinnamon stick and cook, stirring, for 1 minute. Add mushrooms and toss until coated. Add tomatoes with juice and bring to a boil. Transfer to slow cooker stoneware.

NUTRIENTS PER SERVING	
Calories	205
Fat	4.0 g
Saturates	0.5 g
Polyunsaturates	1.0 g
Monounsaturates	2.0 g
Cholesterol	0 mg
Sodium	595 mg
Carbohydrate	38.8 g
Fiber	6.7 g
Protein	7.5 g

AMERICA'S EXCHANGES	
2	Starch
1	Vegetable
½	Fat

CANADA'S CHOICES	
2	Carbohydrate
½	Meat and Alternatives

Make Ahead

This dish can be partially prepared before it is cooked. Complete Step 1. Cover and refrigerate for up to 2 days. When you're ready to cook, continue with the recipe.

2. Add squash and chickpeas and stir well. Cover and cook on Low for 8 hours or on High for 4 hours, until vegetables are tender.

3. In a small bowl, combine honey and lemon juice. Add to slow cooker and stir well.

Mindful Morsels

Mushrooms team up well with numerous other ingredients. In many recipes, I like to use cremini mushrooms for their more intense flavor. One cup (125 mL) of sliced raw mushrooms or $\frac{1}{2}$ cup (125 mL) of cooked mushrooms contains less than 20 calories and almost no fat, is a good source of the B vitamins pantothenic acid and riboflavin, and is a source of the antioxidant mineral selenium. Count these amounts as a Free Food/Extra.

MAKES 10 SERVINGS

Tips

If you prefer, use frozen chopped butternut squash in this recipe. Reduce the quantity to 2 cups (500 mL).

Be sure to rinse the quinoa thoroughly before using because some quinoa has a resinous coating called saponin, which needs to be rinsed off. To ensure your quinoa is saponin-free, before cooking fill a bowl with warm water and swish the kernels around, then transfer to a sieve and rinse thoroughly under cold running water.

Squash with Quinoa and Apricots

Banish the blahs with this robust combination of fruits, vegetables and a nutritious whole grain seasoned with ginger, orange and a hint of cinnamon. In season, garnish with watercress.

• **Works in slow cookers from 3½ to 6 quarts**

1 tbsp	cumin seeds	15 mL
1 tbsp	olive oil	15 mL
2	onions, finely chopped	2
2	cloves garlic, minced	2
1 tbsp	minced gingerroot	15 mL
2 tsp	finely grated orange zest	10 mL
1	piece (2 inches/5 cm) cinnamon stick	1
1 tsp	turmeric	5 mL
1 tsp	salt	5 mL
½ tsp	cracked black peppercorns	2 mL
1 cup	lower-salt vegetable broth	250 mL
½ cup	orange juice	125 mL
4 cups	cubed (1 inch/2.5 cm) peeled squash (see Tips, left)	1 L
2	apples, peeled, cored and sliced	2
½ cup	chopped dried apricots	125 mL
1½ cups	quinoa, rinsed (see Tips, left)	375 mL

1. In a large dry skillet over medium heat, toast cumin seeds, stirring, until fragrant and they just begin to brown, about 3 minutes. Immediately transfer to a mortar or spice grinder and grind. Set aside.

2. In same skillet, heat oil over medium heat for 30 seconds. Add onions and cook, stirring, until softened, about 3 minutes. Add garlic, gingerroot, orange zest, cinnamon stick, turmeric, salt and peppercorns and cook, stirring, for 1 minute. Add broth and orange juice and bring to a boil. Transfer to slow cooker stoneware.

NUTRIENTS PER SERVING	
Calories	185
Fat	3.3 g
Saturates	0.4 g
Polyunsaturates	0.8 g
Monounsaturates	1.5 g
Cholesterol	0 mg
Sodium	318 mg
Carbohydrate	36.6 g
Fiber	4.3 g
Protein	4.7 g

AMERICA'S EXCHANGES	
1½	Starch
1	Fruit

CANADA'S CHOICES	
2	Carbohydrate
½	Fat

This dish can be partially prepared before it is cooked. Complete Steps 1 and 2. Cover and refrigerate overnight or for up to 2 days. When you're ready to cook, continue with Steps 3 and 4.

3. Add squash, apples and apricots to stoneware and stir well. Cover and cook on Low for 6 hours or on High for 3 hours, until vegetables are tender.

4. In a pot, bring 3 cups (750 mL) of water to a boil. Add quinoa in a steady stream, stirring to prevent lumps from forming, and return to a boil. Cover, reduce heat to low and simmer for 15 minutes, until tender and liquid is absorbed. Add to slow cooker and stir well. Serve immediately.

Mindful Morsels

Quinoa is extremely nutritious — so nutritious, in fact, that it's been called a "supergrain." Originally grown in the Andes, this hardy "grain of the Incas" has recently been rediscovered. Unlike wheat and rice, quinoa protein is complete, because it contains lysine. Like all whole grains, it is a source of vitamins, minerals and beneficial phytonutrients.

MAKES 12 SERVINGS

Make Ahead

This dish can be partially prepared before it is cooked. Complete Step 1. Cover and refrigerate overnight or up to 2 days. When you're ready to cook, continue with Step 2.

Pumpkin and Rice Casserole with Mushrooms

This simple casserole makes a nice weeknight dinner. Serve it with a green salad or sliced tomatoes, in season.

- **Large (minimum 5 quart) slow cooker**

1 tbsp	olive oil	15 mL
2	onions, diced	2
2	stalks celery, diced	2
2	carrots, peeled and diced	2
2	cloves garlic, minced	2
1 tsp	dried thyme leaves, crumbled	5 mL
½ tsp	salt	2 mL
½ tsp	cracked black peppercorns	2 mL
12 oz	cremini mushrooms, trimmed and quartered	375 g
2 cups	long-grain brown rice	500 mL
1	can (28 oz/796 mL) diced tomatoes, including juice	1
2 cups	lower-salt vegetable broth	500 mL
4 cups	cubed (½ inch/1 cm) peeled pumpkin or orange or yellow squash	1 L
1	chipotle pepper in adobo sauce, minced	1
2 cups	shredded light Monterey Jack cheese	500 mL

1. In a large skillet, heat oil over medium heat for 30 seconds. Add onions, celery and carrots and cook, stirring, until carrots are softened, about 7 minutes. Add garlic, thyme, salt and peppercorns and cook, stirring, for 1 minute. Add mushrooms and toss to coat. Add rice and toss to coat. Add tomatoes, with juice, and broth and bring to a boil. Transfer to slow cooker stoneware. Stir in pumpkin.

2. Place one clean tea towel, folded in half (so you will have two layers) across the top of slow cooker stoneware, to absorb moisture. Cover and cook on Low for 7 to 8 hours or on High for 4 hours, until rice is tender and liquid is absorbed. Remove tea towel. Stir in chipotle pepper and sprinkle cheese over top of mixture. Cover and cook on High for 20 to 25 minutes, until flavors meld and cheese is melted.

NUTRIENTS PER SERVING	
Calories	231
Fat	6.6 g
Saturates	3.1 g
Polyunsaturates	0.7 g
Monounsaturates	2.3 g
Cholesterol	12 mg
Sodium	409 mg
Carbohydrate	34.2 g
Fiber	4.2 g
Protein	10.0 g

AMERICA'S EXCHANGES	
2	Starch
1	Medium-fat Meat

CANADA'S CHOICES	
2	Carbohydrate
1	Meat and Alternatives

Peas and Greens

MAKES 4 SERVINGS

This delicious combination of black-eyed peas and greens, which is a Greek tradition, is a great dish for busy weeknights. It also makes a wonderful side dish for roasted meat, particularly lamb.

Tips

To toast fennel seeds: Place seeds in a dry skillet over medium heat and cook, stirring, until fragrant and they just begin to brown, about 3 minutes. Immediately transfer to a mortar or a spice grinder and grind. (Or place the seeds on a cutting board and use the bottom of a wine bottle or measuring cup.)

Use any kind of paprika in this recipe. Hot paprika will add the zest heat seekers prefer. Smoked paprika will enhance the flavor with a pleasant smokiness.

Make Ahead

This dish can be partially prepared before it is cooked. Complete Step 1. Cover and refrigerate for up to 2 days. When you're ready to cook, continue with the recipe.

* **Works in slow cookers from 3½ to 6 quarts**

1 tbsp	olive oil	15 mL
2	onions, finely chopped	2
1	bulb fennel, cored, leafy stems discarded, bulb sliced on the vertical	1
4	cloves garlic, minced	4
½ tsp	salt	2 mL
½ tsp	cracked black peppercorns	2 mL
¼ tsp	fennel seeds, toasted and ground (see Tips, left)	1 mL
1	can (14 oz/398 mL) diced tomatoes, including juice	1
2 cups	cooked dried or canned black-eyed peas, drained and rinsed (see Variation, page 231)	500 mL
2 tbsp	freshly squeezed lemon juice	25 mL
1 tsp	paprika (see Tips, left)	5 mL
4 cups	trimmed chopped spinach or Swiss chard (about 1 bunch)	1 L

1. In a skillet, heat oil over medium heat for 30 seconds. Add onions and fennel and cook, stirring, until fennel is softened, about 5 minutes. Add garlic, salt, peppercorns and toasted fennel and cook, stirring, for 1 minute. Add tomatoes with juice and bring to a boil. Transfer to slow cooker stoneware.

2. Add peas and stir well. Cover and cook on Low for 8 hours or on High for 4 hours, until peas are tender. In a small bowl, combine lemon juice and paprika, stirring, until paprika dissolves. Add to slow cooker stoneware and stir well. Add spinach, stirring, until submerged. Cover and cook on High for 20 minutes, until spinach is tender.

NUTRIENTS PER SERVING	
Calories	210
Fat	4.7 g
Saturates	0.7 g
Polyunsaturates	0.8 g
Monounsaturates	2.6 g
Cholesterol	0 mg
Sodium	542 mg
Carbohydrate	34.8 g
Fiber	8.2 g
Protein	11.1 g

AMERICA'S EXCHANGES	
2	Starch
1	Vegetable
½	Lean Meat

CANADA'S CHOICES	
2	Carbohydrate
1	Meat and Alternatives

Red Beans and Greens

MAKES 10 SERVINGS

Make Ahead

This dish can be partially prepared before it is cooked. Complete Steps 1 and 2. Cover and refrigerate for up to 2 days. When you're ready to cook, continue with the recipe.

Few meals could be more healthful than this delicious combination of hot leafy greens and flavorful beans. I like to make this with collard greens, but other dark leafy greens such as kale work well too. The smoked paprika makes the dish more robust, but it isn't essential. If you're cooking for a smaller group, make the full quantity of beans, spoon off what is needed, and serve with the appropriate quantity of cooked greens. Refrigerate or freeze the leftover beans for another meal.

• **Works in slow cookers from 3½ to 6 quarts**

2 cups	dried red kidney beans	500 mL
1 tbsp	olive oil	15 mL
2	large onions, finely chopped	2
2	stalks celery, finely chopped	2
4	cloves garlic, minced	4
1 tsp	dried oregano leaves	5 mL
1 tsp	salt	5 mL
½ tsp	cracked black peppercorns	2 mL
½ tsp	dried thyme leaves	2 mL
¼ tsp	ground allspice or 6 whole allspice (tied in a piece of cheesecloth)	1 mL
2	bay leaves	2
4 cups	lower-salt vegetable broth	1 L
1 tsp	paprika, preferably smoked, optional	5 mL

Greens

2 lbs	greens, such as collards, thoroughly washed, stems removed and leaves chopped	1 kg
1 tbsp	olive oil	15 mL
1 tbsp	balsamic vinegar	15 mL
	Freshly ground black pepper	

1. Soak beans according to either method in Basic Beans (see page 231). Drain and rinse and set aside.

2. In a skillet, heat oil over medium heat for 30 seconds. Add onions and celery and cook, stirring, until softened, about 5 minutes. Add garlic, oregano, salt, peppercorns, thyme, allspice and bay leaves and cook, stirring for 1 minute. Transfer to slow cooker stoneware. Add beans and broth.

NUTRIENTS PER SERVING	
Calories	189
Fat	3.3 g
Saturates	0.4 g
Polyunsaturates	0.4 g
Monounsaturates	2.0 g
Cholesterol	0 mg
Sodium	439 mg
Carbohydrate	30.6 g
Fiber	11.8 g
Protein	11.1 g

AMERICA'S EXCHANGES	
2	Starch
1	Very Lean Meat

CANADA'S CHOICES	
1	Carbohydrate
1	Meat and Alternatives

3. Cover and cook on Low for 8 to 10 hours or on High for 4 to 5 hours, until beans are tender. Stir in smoked paprika, if using.

4. **Greens:** In a large pot or steamer, steam greens until tender, about 10 minutes for collards. Toss with oil and balsamic vinegar. Season to taste with pepper. Add to beans and stir to combine. Serve immediately.

Mindful Morsels

Dried beans package lots of nutrients with relatively few calories and almost no fat. Well known for their fiber content, legumes (dried beans, peas and lentils) offer several other nutritional advantages: $\frac{1}{2}$ cup (125 mL) of prepared dried beans has about 155 calories, 21 g of protein and a generous 8 g of fiber, but only 1 g of sodium (when prepared without salt) and almost no fat. Not many foods are as nutrient-dense as dried beans: $\frac{1}{2}$ cup (125 mL) is an excellent source of folacin and a good source of iron, magnesium and manganese; it also supplies smaller but significant amounts of thiamine, niacin, potassium and zinc. Like other high-fiber foods, beans help fill you up and make it easier to resist overeating.

Greek-Style Beans and Barley

MAKES 8 SERVINGS

Tips

If possible, use golden or yellow zucchini, which has more flavor than the green version. If you're not peeling it, scrub the skin thoroughly with a vegetable brush.

If you prefer, complete Step 3 while the zucchini sweats. When finished, wipe skillet clean and complete Step 2.

Here's a tasty casserole the whole family can enjoy. Add a simple green or shredded carrot salad for a great weekday meal.

- **Works in slow cookers from 3½ to 6 quarts**

2	zucchini, sliced into ½-inch (1 cm) slices (see Tips, left)	2
½ tsp	salt	2 mL
2 tbsp	olive oil, divided	25 mL
4	cloves garlic, minced	4
	Freshly ground black pepper	
2	onions, finely chopped	2
2 tsp	dried oregano leaves, crumbled	10 mL
½ tsp	cracked black peppercorns	2 mL
1	can (28 oz/796 mL) diced tomatoes, including juice	1
2 tbsp	tomato paste	25 mL
2 cups	lower-salt vegetable broth	500 mL
1 cup	pearl, whole (hulled) or pot barley (see Mindful Morsels, opposite)	250 mL
3 cups	frozen sliced green beans	750 mL
½ cup	crumbled light feta cheese, optional	125 mL

1. In a colander over a sink, combine zucchini and salt. Toss well and set aside for 30 minutes to allow zucchini to sweat. Rinse thoroughly. Pat dry with paper towel.

2. In a skillet, heat 1 tbsp (15 mL) of the oil over medium heat for 30 seconds. Add zucchini and cook, stirring, for 3 minutes. Add garlic and cook, stirring, until zucchini softens and just begins to brown, about 4 minutes. Season to taste with freshly ground black pepper. Transfer to a bowl, cover and refrigerate.

3. In same skillet, heat remaining oil over medium heat for 30 seconds. Add onions and cook, stirring, until softened, about 3 minutes. Add oregano and peppercorns and cook, stirring, for 1 minute. Add tomatoes with juice, tomato paste and broth and bring to a boil. Transfer to slow cooker stoneware.

NUTRIENTS PER SERVING	
Calories	170
Fat	4.0 g
Saturates	0.6 g
Polyunsaturates	0.6 g
Monounsaturates	2.6 g
Cholesterol	0 mg
Sodium	299 mg
Carbohydrate	32.2 g
Fiber	5.00 g
Protein	3.8 g

AMERICA'S EXCHANGES	
1	Starch
1	Other Carbohydrate
½	Fat
1	Free Food

CANADA'S CHOICES	
2	Carbohydrate
1	Fat

Make Ahead

This dish can be partially prepared before it is cooked. Complete Steps 1 through 3. Cover and refrigerate separately overnight or for up to 2 days. When you're ready to cook, continue with Step 4.

4. Add barley and green beans and stir well. Cover and cook on Low for 6 hours or on High for 3 hours, until barley is tender. Add reserved zucchini and stir well. Cover and cook on High for 15 minutes, until zucchini is heated through. Sprinkle with crumbled feta, if using.

Mindful Morsels

To boost the nutritional value of this dish, use whole grain (hulled or pot) barley rather than the pearled variety. A $\frac{1}{2}$-cup (125 mL) serving of cooked whole grain barley contains a high amount of dietary fiber and is especially high in soluble fiber, which helps to keep cholesterol under control. It is also a good source of the antioxidant mineral selenium.

New Age Succotash

MAKES 8 SERVINGS

Make Ahead

This dish can be partially prepared before it is cooked. Complete Step 1. Cover and refrigerate overnight or for up to 2 days. When you're ready to cook, continue with Step 2.

Variation

Spicy Succotash: For a livelier dish, stir in 1 can (4.5 oz/127 mL) mild green chiles along with the red peppers.

I call this dish "new age" because it uses edamame, or soybeans, instead of traditional lima beans. I've also bumped up the flavor with paprika, and finished with a smattering of mouthwatering roasted red peppers, usually not included in the dish. I like to serve this with steamed asparagus, in season.

- **Works in slow cookers from 3½ to 6 quarts**

1 tbsp	olive oil	15 mL
2	onions, finely chopped	2
4	stalks celery, diced	4
2	carrots, peeled and diced	2
4	cloves garlic, minced	4
1	sprig fresh rosemary or 2 tsp (10 mL) dried rosemary leaves, crumbled	1
½ tsp	salt	2 mL
½ tsp	cracked black peppercorns	2 mL
1	can (28 oz/796 mL) diced tomatoes, including juice	1
1½ cups	lower-salt vegetable broth	375 mL
4 cups	frozen shelled edamame	1 L
4 cups	frozen corn kernels	1 L
2 tsp	paprika, dissolved in 2 tbsp (25 mL) water	10 mL
2	roasted red bell peppers, diced	2
½ cup	finely chopped parsley leaves	125 mL

1. In a skillet, heat oil over medium heat for 30 seconds. Add onions, celery and carrots and cook, stirring, until softened, about 7 minutes. Add garlic, rosemary, salt and peppercorns and cook, stirring, for 1 minute. Stir in tomatoes with juices and broth and bring to a boil. Transfer to slow cooker stoneware.

2. Add edamame and corn. Stir well. Cover and cook on Low for 8 to 10 hours or on High for 4 to 5 hours, until mixture is hot and bubbly. Stir in paprika solution, roasted red peppers and parsley. Cover and cook on High for 15 minutes, until heated through.

NUTRIENTS PER SERVING	
Calories	324
Fat	11.1 g
Saturates	1.3 g
Polyunsaturates	5.3 g
Monounsaturates	2.4 g
Cholesterol	0 mg
Sodium	530 mg
Carbohydrate	42.9 g
Fiber	9.8 g
Protein	20.9 g

AMERICA'S EXCHANGES	
2	Starch
2	Vegetable
2	Medium-fat Meat

CANADA'S CHOICES	
2	Carbohydrate
2	Meat and Alternatives

MAKES 6 SERVINGS

Tips

You can purchase wild and brown rice mixtures in many supermarkets, or you can make your own by combining ½ cup (125 mL) of each.

Accumulated moisture affects the consistency of the rice. The folded tea towels will absorb the moisture generated during cooking.

Make Ahead

This dish can be partially prepared before it is cooked. Complete Step 1. Cover and refrigerate overnight. The next morning, continue with the recipe.

Wild Rice with Mushrooms and Apricots

This combination of wild and brown rice with dried apricots makes a tasty weeknight meal. Be sure to serve it with a good chutney alongside — tomato or spicy mango work very well. A grated carrot salad is a nice accompaniment.

- **Works in slow cookers from 3½ to 6 quarts**
- **Greased slow cooker stoneware**

1 tbsp	olive oil	15 mL
1	onion, chopped	1
4	stalks celery, diced	4
2	cloves garlic, minced	2
1 cup	wild rice and brown rice mixture, rinsed (see Tips, left)	250 mL
2 cups	lower-salt vegetable broth	500 mL
1 tbsp	balsamic vinegar	15 mL
	Freshly ground black pepper	
8 oz	portobello or cremini mushrooms, stems removed and caps diced	250 g
¼ cup	chopped dried apricots	50 mL
	Chutney	

1. In a skillet, heat oil over medium heat for 30 seconds. Add onion and celery and cook, stirring, until softened, about 5 minutes. Add garlic and rice and stir until coated. Add broth and balsamic vinegar and bring to a boil. Season to taste with pepper. Transfer to prepared stoneware.

2. Stir in mushrooms and apricots. Place two clean tea towels, each folded in half (so you will have four layers), over top of slow cooker stoneware (see Tips, left). Cover and cook on Low for 7 to 8 hours or on High for 3½ to 4 hours, until rice is tender and liquid has been absorbed. Serve hot accompanied by your favorite fruit chutney.

NUTRIENTS PER SERVING	
Calories	181
Fat	3.5 g
Saturates	0.5 g
Polyunsaturates	0.6 g
Monounsaturates	2.0 g
Cholesterol	0 mg
Sodium	182 mg
Carbohydrate	34.2 g
Fiber	3.8 g
Protein	4.7 g

AMERICA'S EXCHANGES	
1½	Starch
1	Vegetable
½	Fruit

CANADA'S CHOICES	
2	Carbohydrate
1	Fat

MAKES 8 SERVINGS

Tip

To toast bread cubes, place on a rimmed baking sheet in a 325°F (160°C) oven for 5 to 7 minutes, stirring twice.

Artichoke, Sun-Dried Tomato and Goat Cheese Strata

This is a great brunch dish. I like to serve it with a green salad.

- **Large (minimum 5 quart) slow cooker**
- **Greased slow cooker stoneware**

8 cups	cubed (½ inch/1 cm) toasted sourdough or whole wheat bread (see Tip, left)	2 L
1 cup	sliced green onions, white part with just a bit of green	250 mL
4 to 6	oil-packed sun-dried tomatoes, drained and finely chopped	4 to 6
1	can (14 oz/398 mL) artichoke hearts, drained and chopped	1
8 oz	soft goat cheese, crumbled, divided	250 g
4	eggs	4
2 cups	2% evaporated milk	500 mL
½ tsp	salt	2 mL
½ tsp	cracked black peppercorns	2 mL

1. In prepared stoneware, combine bread, green onions, sun-dried tomatoes, artichokes and half of the goat cheese. Toss well.

2. In a bowl, whisk together eggs, milk, salt and peppercorns. Pour over bread mixture. Sprinkle remaining goat cheese evenly over top.

3. Place two clean tea towels, each folded in half (so you will have four layers) over top of stoneware to absorb moisture. Cover and cook on Low for 6 hours or on High for 3 hours, until strata is set and edges are browning.

NUTRIENTS PER SERVING	
Calories	280
Fat	11.1 g
Saturates	5.9 g
Polyunsaturates	0.9 g
Monounsaturates	3.3 g
Cholesterol	111 mg
Sodium	663 mg
Carbohydrate	28.3 g
Fiber	3.1 g
Protein	17.2 g

AMERICA'S EXCHANGES	
1	Starch
1	Vegetable
½	Low-fat Milk
1	Lean Meat
1	Fat

CANADA'S CHOICES	
1½	Carbohydrate
1½	Meat and Alternatives
1	Fat

MAKES 4 SERVINGS

Soy-Braised Tofu

It's amazing how tofu soaks up the mouthwatering Asian flavors in this recipe. Use this hot braised tofu as a centerpiece to a meal of vegetarian dishes that might include stir-fried bok choy or wilted greens garnished with toasted sesame seeds. Refrigerate any leftovers for use in other dishes, such as stir-fried mixed vegetables, or salads, such as an Asian-inspired coleslaw. You can also transform this flavorful tofu into a wrap. Place on lettuce leaves, garnish with shredded carrots and fold.

Tip

To drain tofu, place a layer of paper towels on a plate. Set tofu in the middle. Cover with another layer of paper towel and a heavy plate. Set aside for 30 minutes. Peel off paper and cut tofu into cubes.

- **Large (minimum 6 quart) slow cooker**

¼ cup	light (reduced-sodium) soy sauce	50 mL
1 tbsp	puréed gingerroot	15 mL
1 tbsp	pure maple syrup	15 mL
1 tbsp	toasted sesame oil	15 mL
1 tbsp	freshly squeezed lemon juice	15 mL
1 tsp	minced garlic	5 mL
½ tsp	cracked black peppercorns	2 mL
1 lb	firm tofu, drained and cut into 1-inch (2.5 cm) cubes (see Tip, left)	500 g

1. In slow cooker stoneware, combine soy sauce, gingerroot, maple syrup, toasted sesame oil, lemon juice, garlic and peppercorns. Add tofu and toss gently until coated on all sides. Cover and refrigerate for 1 hour.

2. Toss well. Cover and cook on Low for 5 hours or on High for 2½ hours, until tofu is hot and has absorbed the flavor.

Mindful Morsels

Soybeans, from which tofu is made, contain all nine essential amino acids, which means they are a complete protein.

NUTRIENTS PER SERVING	
Calories	144
Fat	8.5 g
Saturates	1.2 g
Polyunsaturates	4.3 g
Monounsaturates	2.5 g
Cholesterol	0 mg
Sodium	610 mg
Carbohydrate	9.3 g
Fiber	1.3 g
Protein	10.2 g

AMERICA'S EXCHANGES	
½	Starch
1	Lean Meat
1	Fat

CANADA'S CHOICES	
½	Carbohydrate
1	Meat and Alternatives
½	Fat

Tofu in Indian-Spiced Tomato Sauce

MAKES 6 SERVINGS

Make Ahead

This dish can be partially prepared before it is cooked. Complete Step 1. Cover and refrigerate for up to 2 days. When you're ready to cook, continue with the recipe.

This robust dish makes a lively and different meal. I like to serve it with fresh green beans and naan, an Indian bread, to soak up the sauce.

• **Works in slow cookers from 3½ to 6 quarts**

1 tbsp	olive oil	15 mL
2	onions, finely chopped	2
2	cloves garlic, minced	2
½ tsp	minced gingerroot	2 mL
6	whole cloves	6
4	pods white or green cardamom	4
1	piece (2 inches/5 cm) cinnamon stick	1
1 tsp	caraway seeds	5 mL
1 tsp	salt	5 mL
½ tsp	cracked black peppercorns	2 mL
1	can (28 oz/796 mL) diced tomatoes, including juice	1
1	long green chile pepper, seeded and finely chopped	1

Tofu

¼ cup	all-purpose flour	50 mL
1 tsp	curry powder	5 mL
¼ tsp	cayenne pepper	1 mL
8 oz	firm tofu, cut into 1-inch (2.5 cm) squares	250 g
1 tbsp	olive oil	15 mL

1. In a skillet, heat oil over medium heat for 30 seconds. Add onions and cook, stirring, until softened, about 3 minutes. Add garlic, gingerroot, cloves, cardamom, cinnamon stick, caraway seeds, salt and peppercorns and cook, stirring, for 1 minute. Add tomatoes with juice and bring to a boil. Transfer to slow cooker stoneware.

2. Cover and cook on Low for 8 hours or on High for 4 hours, until hot and bubbly. Stir in chile pepper.

3. **Tofu:** On a plate, mix together flour, curry powder and cayenne. Roll tofu in mixture until lightly coated. Discard excess flour mixture. In a skillet, heat oil over medium-high heat for 30 seconds. Add dredged tofu and sauté, stirring, until nicely browned. Spoon tomato mixture into a serving dish. Discard cloves, cardamom and cinnamon stick. Layer tofu on top.

NUTRIENTS PER SERVING	
Calories	130
Fat	6.8 g
Saturates	0.9 g
Polyunsaturates	1.5 g
Monounsaturates	3.8 g
Cholesterol	0 mg
Sodium	614 mg
Carbohydrate	14.4 g
Fiber	2.1 g
Protein	5.4 g

AMERICA'S EXCHANGES	
½	Starch
1	Vegetable
½	Lean Meat
1	Fat

CANADA'S CHOICES	
1	Carbohydrate
½	Meat and Alternatives
1	Fat

Fish and Seafood

Tips

Large cans of tomatoes come in 28 oz (796 mL) and 35 oz (980 mL) sizes. For convenience, I've called for the 28 oz (796 mL) size in my recipes. If you're using the 35 oz (980 mL) size, drain off 1 cup (250 mL) liquid before adding to the recipe.

Chile nomenclature can be confusing. Long green chiles are usually used in Indian cooking and can be found in Asian markets. They are sometimes called cayenne or serrano chiles, not to be confused with Mexican serrano chiles, which are different.

Halibut in Indian-Spiced Tomato Sauce

This robust fish recipe is almost a meal in itself. I like to serve it with fresh green beans and naan, an Indian bread, to soak up the sauce.

- **Works in slow cookers from 3½ to 6 quarts**

2 tbsp	olive oil, divided	25 mL
2	onions, finely chopped	2
2	cloves garlic, minced	2
½ tsp	minced gingerroot	2 mL
2	whole cloves	2
2	white or green cardamom pods	2
1	piece (2 inches/5 cm) cinnamon stick	1
½ tsp	caraway seeds	2 mL
1 tsp	salt	5 mL
½ tsp	cracked black peppercorns	2 mL
1	can (28 oz/796 mL) diced tomatoes, including juice (see Tips, left)	1
2	potatoes, peeled and diced	2
1	long green chile pepper, seeded and finely chopped (see Tips, left)	1
¼ cup	all-purpose flour	50 mL
1 tsp	turmeric	5 mL
½ tsp	ground coriander	2 mL
¼ tsp	cayenne pepper	1 mL
1½ lbs	halibut fillets, cut into 1-inch (2.5 cm) squares	750 g

1. In a skillet, heat 1 tbsp (15 mL) of the oil over medium heat for 30 seconds. Add onions and cook, stirring, until softened, about 3 minutes. Add garlic, gingerroot, cloves, cardamom, cinnamon stick, caraway seeds, salt and peppercorns and cook, stirring, for 1 minute. Add tomatoes with juice and bring to a boil. Transfer to slow cooker stoneware.

2. Add potatoes and stir well. Cover and cook on Low for 8 to 10 hours or on High for 4 to 5 hours, until potatoes are tender. Stir in chile pepper.

NUTRIENTS PER SERVING	
Calories	192
Fat	5.8 g
Saturates	0.8 g
Polyunsaturates	1.1 g
Monounsaturates	3.2 g
Cholesterol	27 mg
Sodium	505 mg
Carbohydrate	15.3 g
Fiber	1.8 g
Protein	20.0 g

AMERICA'S EXCHANGES	
½	Starch
1½	Vegetable
2	Lean Meat

CANADA'S CHOICES	
1	Carbohydrate
2½	Meat and Alternatives

Make Ahead

This dish can be partially prepared before it is cooked. Complete Step 1. Cover and refrigerate for up to 2 days. When you're ready to cook, continue with the recipe.

3. On a plate, mix together flour, turmeric, coriander and cayenne. Roll halibut in mixture until lightly coated. Discard excess flour. In a skillet, heat remaining oil over medium-high heat for 30 seconds. Add dredged halibut and sauté, in batches if necessary, stirring, until fish is nicely browned and cooked to desired doneness. Spoon tomato mixture into a serving dish and layer halibut on top.

Mindful Morsels

Onions are the base for so many soups, stews and sauces that we take them for granted. But onions contain many nutrients, including the flavonoid quercitin. A study published in the *American Journal of Clinical Nutrition* in 2002 linked a high intake of flavonoids with a lower incidence of heart disease and stroke.

Make Ahead

This dish can be prepared before it is cooked. Complete Steps 1 through 3. Cover and refrigerate overnight. When you're ready to cook, continue with Step 4.

Variation

Dill Salmon Loaf: Substitute ½ tsp (2 mL) dried dillweed or thyme for tarragon and ½ cup (125 mL) chopped dill for parsley.

Salmon Loaf

This tasty loaf, accompanied by a tossed green salad, is a favorite weekday meal at our house. If you don't have tomato sauce, homemade chili sauce or another tomato-based relish also makes a nice finish. Or try a yogurt-based sauce such as tzatziki.

• **Works in slow cookers from 3½ to 6 quarts**

1 tbsp	olive oil	15 mL
1	large onion, finely chopped (about 1½ cups/375 mL)	1
4	stalks celery, finely chopped (about 1½ cups/375 mL)	4
8 oz	mushrooms, thinly sliced	250 g
½ tsp	dried tarragon, crumbled	2 mL
½ tsp	freshly ground black pepper	2 mL
3	eggs	3
2 tbsp	freshly squeezed lemon juice	25 mL
2	cans (each 7½ oz/213 g) wild salmon, including bones and juice, skin removed, if desired	2
½ cup	finely chopped parsley	125 mL
¾ cup	dry bread crumbs (approx.)	175 mL
	Warm tomato sauce, optional	

1. In a skillet, heat oil over medium heat for 30 seconds. Add onion, celery and mushrooms and cook, stirring, until celery is tender, about 5 minutes. Add tarragon and pepper and cook, stirring, for 1 minute. Remove from heat and set aside.

2. In a bowl large enough to accommodate salmon and vegetables, beat eggs and lemon juice. Add salmon with bones and juice and break into small pieces with a fork. Add reserved mushroom mixture, parsley and bread crumbs and mix until blended. If mixture still seems wet, add more bread crumbs, 1 tbsp (15 mL) at a time, until liquid is absorbed.

NUTRIENTS PER SERVING	
Calories	247
Fat	12.9 g
Saturates	2.9 g
Polyunsaturates	2.1 g
Monounsaturates	5.2 g
Cholesterol	111 mg
Sodium	467 mg
Carbohydrate	14.7 g
Fiber	1.7 g
Protein	17.9 g

AMERICA'S EXCHANGES	
1	Starch
2	Lean Meat
1½	Fat

CANADA'S CHOICES	
1	Carbohydrate
2	Meat and Alternatives
1	Fat

If you prefer and you have a large oval slow cooker, you can make this in an 8- by 4-inch (20 by 10 cm) loaf pan, lightly greased. You won't need the foil strip, but you will need to cover the pan tightly with foil after filling it with the salmon mixture. Then the foil should be secured with a string or elastic band. Place the pan in the slow cooker stoneware and pour in enough boiling water to come 1 inch (2.5 cm) up the sides. Cover and cook on Low for 6 hours or on High for 3 hours, or until loaf is set.

3. Fold a 2-foot (60 cm) piece of foil in half lengthwise. Place on bottom and up the sides of slow cooker stoneware (see Tip, left). Shape salmon mixture into a loaf and place in middle of foil strip on bottom of slow cooker stoneware.

4. Cover and cook on Low for 4 to 5 hours or on High for 2 to $2\frac{1}{2}$ hours, or until loaf is set. Slide the loaf off the foil onto a platter and slice. Top with a dollop of tomato sauce, if using.

Mindful Morsels

Every cell in our bodies needs omega-3 fatty acids to build strong cell membranes. And studies indicate that these fatty acids, found primarily in coldwater fish and some vegetable oils, also appear to reduce the risk of coronary heart disease and other chronic diseases. Salmon is one of the best sources of omega-3 fatty acids.

Tips

Make sure that the salmon is completely covered with the poaching liquid. If you do not have sufficient liquid, add water to cover.

When the salmon is cooked, it should feel firm to the touch and the skin should peel off easily.

Make Ahead

You can make the poaching liquid before you intend to cook. Cover and refrigerate for up to 2 days.

Poached Salmon

Although I love salmon cooked almost any way, poaching produces the moistest result. The problem is, successfully poaching a large piece of salmon used to require a fish poacher, a piece of kitchen equipment that was rarely used yet relatively costly and cumbersome to store. A large oval slow cooker is the ideal solution. It produces great results with little fuss. Serve poached salmon, warm or cold, as the focus of an elegant buffet or dinner, attractively garnished with sliced lemon and sprigs of parsley or dill, and accompany with your favorite sauce.

• **Works best in a large (minimum 5 quart) oval slow cooker**

Poaching Liquid

6 cups	water	1.5 L
1	onion, chopped	1
2	stalks celery, chopped, or $\frac{1}{2}$ tsp (2 mL) celery seeds	2
4	sprigs parsley	4
$\frac{1}{2}$ cup	white wine or freshly squeezed lemon juice	125 mL
8	whole black peppercorns	8
1	bay leaf	1

Salmon

1	fillet of salmon (about 3 lbs/1.5 kg)	1
	Lemon slices	
	Sprigs fresh parsley or dill	

1. **Poaching Liquid:** In a saucepan, combine water, onion, celery, parsley, white wine, peppercorns and bay leaf over medium heat. Bring to a boil and simmer for 30 minutes. Strain and discard solids.

2. **Salmon:** Preheat slow cooker on High for 15 minutes. Fold a 2-foot (60 cm) piece of foil in half lengthwise. Place on bottom and up sides of stoneware, allowing it to overhang the casing a bit. Lay salmon over foil strip. Return poaching liquid to a boil and pour over salmon (see Tips, left). Cover and cook on High for 1 hour. Remove stoneware from slow cooker. Allow salmon to cool in stoneware for 20 minutes. If serving cold, place stoneware in refrigerator and allow salmon to chill in liquid. When cold, lift out and transfer to a platter. If serving hot, lift out and transfer to a platter. Garnish with lemon slices and sprigs of parsley and serve.

NUTRIENTS PER SERVING	
Calories	151
Fat	9.1 g
Saturates	1.8 g
Polyunsaturates	3.3 g
Monounsaturates	3.3 g
Cholesterol	46 mg
Sodium	45 mg
Carbohydrate	0.0 g
Fiber	0.0 g
Protein	16.2 g

AMERICA'S EXCHANGES	
2	Medium-fat Meat

CANADA'S CHOICES	
2	Meat and Alternatives

Tips

Large cans of tomatoes come in 28 oz (796 mL) and 35 oz (980 mL) sizes. For convenience, I've called for the 28 oz (796 mL) size in my recipes.

If you use tortillas with this dish, count a 6- to 7-inch (15 to 18 cm) tortilla as 1 Starch Exchange or 1 Carbohydrate Choice plus 1/2 Fat Choice.

Make Ahead

This dish can be partially prepared before it is cooked. Complete Step 1. Cover and refrigerate mixture for up to 2 days. When you're ready to cook, continue with the recipe.

Snapper Vera Cruz

This traditional Mexican recipe has many variations. Most often, filleted fish is fried and covered with a sauce that is cooked separately. For this slow cooker version, I've sliced the fish very thinly and poached it in the sauce during the last 20 minutes of cooking. For an authentic Mexican touch, serve with hot tortillas to soak up the sauce. Feel free to use any firm white fish instead of snapper.

• **Works in slow cookers from 3 1/2 to 6 quarts**

1 tbsp	olive oil	15 mL
1	onion, finely chopped	1
2	cloves garlic, minced	2
1/2 tsp	dried oregano leaves	2 mL
1/4 tsp	ground cinnamon	1 mL
1/8 tsp	ground cloves	0.5 mL
1	can (28 oz/796 mL) diced tomatoes, drained (see Tips, left)	1
1/2 cup	fish stock or bottled clam juice	125 mL
1 1/2 lbs	skinless snapper fillets, cut in half lengthwise and sliced as thinly as possible on the horizontal	750 g
1 to 2	jalapeño peppers, finely chopped	1 to 2
2 tbsp	freshly squeezed lemon juice	25 mL
1 tbsp	drained capers	15 mL
10	olives, pitted and thinly sliced	10
	Hot whole wheat tortillas, optional	

1. In a skillet, heat oil over medium heat for 30 seconds. Add onion and cook, stirring, until softened, about 3 minutes. Add garlic, oregano, cinnamon and cloves and cook, stirring, for 1 minute. Add tomatoes and stock and bring to a boil. Transfer to slow cooker stoneware.

2. Cover and cook on Low for 6 hours or on High for 3 hours, until hot and bubbly. Stir in fish, jalapeño peppers and lemon juice. Cover and cook on High for 20 minutes, or until fish is cooked through. Stir in capers and pour mixture onto a deep platter. Garnish with olives and serve with hot tortillas, if desired.

NUTRIENTS PER SERVING	
Calories	127
Fat	3.5 g
Saturates	0.6 g
Polyunsaturates	0.7 g
Monounsaturates	1.8 g
Cholesterol	31 mg
Sodium	251 mg
Carbohydrate	5.2 g
Fiber	1.0 g
Protein	18.4 g

AMERICA'S EXCHANGES	
1	Vegetable
2 1/2	Very Lean Meat

CANADA'S CHOICES	
2 1/2	Meat and Alternatives

Tips

For added fiber, use whole wheat pasta.

Make Ahead

This recipe can be assembled before it is cooked. Complete Steps 1 and 2. Cover and refrigerate overnight. When you're ready to cook, continue with Steps 3 and 4.

Creamy Tuna Casserole

In this family-friendly dish, tuna is combined with pasta, mushrooms and other vegetables in a delectable creamy base. The Crispy Crumb Topping adds crunch and a bit of punch in the form of Parmesan cheese. Serve with a tossed green salad for a tasty and nutritious meal.

- **Works in slow cookers from 3½ to 6 quarts**
- **Greased slow cooker stoneware**

8 oz	small tubular pasta, such as penne	250 g
1 tbsp	olive oil	15 mL
1	onion, minced	1
4	stalks celery, diced	4
8 oz	mushrooms, sliced	250 g
½ tsp	dried tarragon or thyme leaves, crumbled	2 mL
½ tsp	cracked black peppercorns	2 mL
1	can (10 oz/284 mL) reduced-salt condensed cream of mushroom soup, undiluted	1
2 tbsp	light cream cheese, softened	25 mL
2	cans (each 6 oz/170 g) solid white tuna, drained and flaked	2

Crispy Crumb Topping

1 tbsp	butter	15 mL
½ tsp	salt	2 mL
2 cups	fresh bread crumbs	500 mL
2 tbsp	freshly grated Parmesan cheese	25 mL

1. In a pot of boiling salted water, cook pasta until tender to the bite, about 8 minutes. Drain and transfer to prepared slow cooker stoneware.

2. Meanwhile, in a large skillet, heat oil over medium heat for 30 seconds. Add onion, celery and mushrooms and cook, stirring, until celery is softened, about 6 minutes. Add tarragon and peppercorns and stir well. Gradually add soup, stirring to dissolve any lumps. Add cream cheese and cook, stirring, until melted and incorporated into sauce. Stir in tuna. Transfer to slow cooker stoneware. Stir well.

3. Cover and cook on Low for 4 to 5 hours or on High for 2 to 2½ hours, until hot and bubbly.

4. **Crispy Crumb Topping:** In a skillet over medium heat, melt butter and salt. Add bread crumbs and cook, stirring, until they start to brown, about 5 minutes. Remove from heat and stir in Parmesan. Spread evenly over top of the cooked casserole and serve.

NUTRIENTS PER SERVING	
Calories	259
Fat	6.7 g
Saturates	2.4 g
Polyunsaturates	0.9 g
Monounsaturates	2.5 g
Cholesterol	22 mg
Sodium	229 mg
Carbohydrate	34.9 g
Fiber	2.8 g
Protein	14.6 g

AMERICA'S EXCHANGES	
2	Starch
1	Vegetable
1	Lean Meat

CANADA'S CHOICES	
2	Carbohydrate
1	Meat and Alternatives
½	Fat

Caribbean Fish Stew

I love the combination of flavors in this tasty stew. The allspice and the Scotch bonnet peppers add a distinctly island tang. For a distinctive and delicious finish, be sure to include the dill. Serve this with crusty rolls to soak up the sauce, a fresh green salad and some crisp white wine.

Tip

One Scotch bonnet pepper is probably enough for most people, but if you're a heat seeker, use two. You can also use habanero pepper equally sparingly instead.

Make Ahead

This dish can be partially prepared before it is cooked. Complete Steps 1 and 2. Cover and refrigerate overnight or for up to 2 days. When you're ready to cook, continue with Step 3.

• **Works in slow cookers from 3½ to 6 quarts**

2 tsp	cumin seeds	10 mL
6	whole allspice	6
1 tbsp	olive oil	15 mL
2	onions, finely chopped	2
4	cloves garlic, minced	4
2 tsp	dried thyme leaves, crumbled	10 mL
1 tsp	turmeric	5 mL
1 tbsp	grated orange or lime zest	15 mL
½ tsp	cracked black peppercorns	2 mL
1	can (28 oz/796 mL) diced tomatoes, including juice	1
2 cups	fish stock	500 mL
1 to 2	Scotch bonnet peppers, minced	1 to 2
2 cups	sliced okra (¼-inch/0.5 cm slices)	500 mL
1½ lbs	skinless grouper fillets, cut into bite-size pieces	750 g
8 oz	shrimp, cooked, peeled and deveined (see Tips, page 148)	250 g
½ cup	finely chopped dill, optional	125 mL

1. In a large dry skillet over medium heat, toast cumin seeds and allspice, stirring, until fragrant and cumin seeds just begin to brown, about 3 minutes. Immediately transfer to a mortar or a spice grinder and grind. Set aside.

2. In same skillet, heat oil over medium heat for 30 seconds. Add onions and cook, stirring, until softened, about 3 minutes. Add garlic, thyme, turmeric, orange zest, peppercorns and reserved cumin and allspice and cook, stirring, for 1 minute. Add tomatoes, with juice, and fish stock and bring to a boil. Transfer to slow cooker stoneware.

3. Cover and cook on Low for 6 hours or on High for 3 hours. Add Scotch bonnet peppers, okra, fish fillets and shrimp. Cover and cook on High for 20 minutes, until fish flakes easily with a fork and okra is tender. Stir in dill, if using.

NUTRIENTS PER SERVING

Calories	138
Fat	3.0 g
Saturates	0.6 g
Polyunsaturates	0.6 g
Monounsaturates	1.4 g
Cholesterol	51 mg
Sodium	294 mg
Carbohydrate	8.4 g
Fiber	1.9 g
Protein	19.4 g

AMERICA'S EXCHANGES

1½	Vegetable
2½	Very Lean Meat

CANADA'S CHOICES

½	Carbohydrate
2½	Meat and Alternatives

Tips

Canned tomatoes vary in sizes. If your supermarket carries the 19-oz (540 mL) can of diced tomatoes, by all means substitute it in this recipe.

If you don't like clams, you can substitute an equal quantity of shucked oysters with their liquid, cooked crabmeat or sliced turkey kielbasa.

Regular blended chili powder works fine in this recipe, but if you prefer you can substitute ancho or New Mexico chili powder or a "gourmet" blend of your choice.

Filé powder, made from dried sassafras leaves, is traditionally used for thickening gumbo. You can find it in specialty food shops.

Louisiana Seafood Stew with Chicken and Sausage

This tasty dish is a variation on gumbo, with less broth and minus the heavy roux for thickening. Gumbo is a bit of a grab bag — within the flavor profile, you can add just about anything. The more health-conscious you are, the more you should downplay sausage and emphasize seafood. This is a rich dish — it just needs rice and a simple green salad to complete the meal.

- **Large (minimum 5 quart) slow cooker**

1 to 2 tbsp	olive oil, divided (approx.)	15 to 25 mL
3 oz	sweet Italian sausage, casings removed and meat crumbled (about 1)	90 g
2	onions, diced	2
4	stalks celery, diced	4
4	cloves garlic, minced	4
1 tsp	dried thyme leaves	5 mL
1 tsp	dried oregano leaves	5 mL
½ tsp	cracked black peppercorns	2 mL
1 tbsp	tomato paste	15 mL
1 tbsp	all-purpose flour	15 mL
3 cups	lower-salt chicken broth	750 mL
1	can (14 oz/398 mL) diced tomatoes, including juice (see Tips, left)	1
1 lb	boneless skinless chicken thighs, cut into bite-size pieces (about 8 thighs)	500 g
8 oz	medium shrimp, cooked, peeled and deveined (see Tips, page 148)	250 g
1	can (5 oz/142 g) clams, drained	1
1	green bell pepper, diced	1
1	red bell pepper, diced	1
½ cup	finely chopped parsley leaves	125 mL
1 tsp	chili powder (see Tips, left)	5 mL
Pinch	cayenne pepper	Pinch
8 oz	sea scallops, halved	250 g
1 tbsp	butter	15 mL
1 tbsp	filé powder, optional (see Tips, left)	15 mL
	Hot pepper sauce	

NUTRIENTS PER SERVING	
Calories	198
Fat	8.4 g
Saturates	2.4 g
Polyunsaturates	1.3 g
Monounsaturates	4.0 g
Cholesterol	94 mg
Sodium	418 mg
Carbohydrate	8.9 g
Fiber	1.8 g
Protein	21.5 g

AMERICA'S EXCHANGES	
1	Vegetable
3	Lean Meat

CANADA'S CHOICES	
½	Carbohydrate
3	Meat and Alternatives

Make Ahead

This dish can be partially prepared before it is cooked. Complete Steps 1 and 2. Cover and refrigerate overnight or for up to 2 days. When you're ready to cook, continue with Steps 3 and 4.

1. In a skillet, heat 1 tbsp (15 mL) of the oil over medium heat. Add sausage and cook, stirring, until no longer pink inside, about 4 minutes. Transfer to slow cooker stoneware.

2. Add remaining oil to pan, if necessary. Add onions and celery and cook, stirring, until celery is tender, about 5 minutes. Add garlic, thyme, oregano and peppercorns and cook, stirring, for 1 minute. Stir in tomato paste. Add flour and cook, stirring, for 1 minute. Add broth and tomatoes with juice and bring to a boil. Cook, stirring, until slightly thickened, about 3 minutes. Transfer to slow cooker stoneware.

3. Add chicken and stir well. Cover and cook on Low for 6 hours or on High for 3 hours, until juices run clear. Add shrimp, clams, green and red peppers and parsley and stir well. Cover and cook on High for 30 minutes, until peppers are tender and shrimp are heated through.

4. Meanwhile, combine chili powder and cayenne in a plastic bag. Add scallops and toss until coated with mixture. In a skillet over medium heat, melt butter. Add scallops and cook, stirring, just until they become opaque, about 4 minutes. Add to slow cooker stoneware and stir well. Add filé powder, if using, and stir well. Serve immediately. Pass the hot pepper sauce at the table.

Tips

To toast fennel seeds: Place seeds in a dry skillet over medium heat, stirring, until fragrant, about 3 minutes. Immediately transfer to a mortar or a spice grinder and grind.

If you don't have fresh thyme, you can use ½ tsp (2 mL) dried thyme. Add it to the recipe in Step 2, along with the garlic.

New World Bouillabaisse

Traditional bouillabaisse contains a wide variety of Mediterranean fish, which leads many to conclude that it can only be made in proximity to the Mediterranean Sea. But in my opinion, this elevates the dish to a status that defies its origins. Bouillabaisse was originally a one-pot meal fishermen made from their daily catch. This simple stew is distinguished by the inclusion of saffron, and a rapid reduction of the broth, which intensifies the flavor and emulsifies the olive oil. Serve this delicious meal-in-a bowl in soup plates, followed by a simple salad and fresh fruit for dessert.

- **Works best in a large (minimum 5 quart) slow cooker**
- **Large square of cheesecloth**

3 tbsp	olive oil, divided	45 mL
1 tsp	fennel seeds, toasted and ground (see Tips, left)	5 mL
1 lb	medium shrimp, peeled and deveined	500 g
1 lb	halibut, cut into 1-inch (2.5 cm) cubes	500 g
2	onions, chopped	2
2	carrots, peeled and diced	2
1	large bulb fennel, cored and thinly sliced on the vertical	1
6	cloves garlic, minced	6
1 tsp	salt	5 mL
½ tsp	cracked black peppercorns	2 mL
1	can (28 oz/796 mL) diced tomatoes, including juice	1
2	potatoes, peeled and diced	2
4 cups	water	1 L
2 cups	dry white wine	500 mL
2 lbs	fish trimmings	1 kg
4	sprigs parsley	4
2	sprigs fresh thyme (see Tips, left)	2
2	bay leaves	2
1 tsp	saffron threads, dissolved in 1 tbsp (15 mL) boiling water	5 mL
24	mussels, cleaned	24
	Crostini (see Tip, opposite)	

Rouille

¼ cup	light mayonnaise	50 mL
1	roasted red pepper, peeled and chopped	1
2	cloves garlic minced	2
Pinch	cayenne pepper	Pinch

NUTRIENTS PER SERVING	
Calories	176
Fat	5.6 g
Saturates	0.8 g
Polyunsaturates	1.0 g
Monounsaturates	3.0 g
Cholesterol	77 mg
Sodium	471 mg
Carbohydrate	12.0 g
Fiber	2.0 g
Protein	19.3 g

AMERICA'S EXCHANGES	
2	Vegetable
2½	Very Lean Meat
½	Fat

CANADA'S CHOICES	
½	Carbohydrate
2½	Meat and Alternatives

To make crostini: Preheat broiler. Brush baguette slices on both sides with olive oil and toast under broiler, turning once.

1. In a bowl, combine 2 tbsp (25 mL) of the olive oil and toasted fennel seeds. Add shrimp and halibut and toss until coated. Cover and refrigerate for 2 hours or overnight, stirring occasionally.

2. In a skillet, heat remaining oil over medium heat for 30 seconds. Add onions, carrots and fennel and cook, stirring, until carrots are softened, about 7 minutes. Add garlic, salt and peppercorns and cook, stirring, for 1 minute. Add tomatoes with juice and bring to a boil. Transfer to slow cooker stoneware.

3. Add potatoes, water and wine to slow cooker and stir well. In a large square of cheesecloth, tie fish trimmings, parsley, thyme and bay leaves. Place in stoneware, ensuring all or most is submerged in the sauce. Cover and cook on Low for 8 to 10 hours or on High for 4 to 5 hours, until vegetables are very tender. Remove package of fish trimmings and discard.

4. Place a colander over a large saucepan and add the soup. Transfer solids to a food processor and purée. Bring liquids in saucepan to a boil over medium-high heat and cook until reduced by about one-third, about 10 minutes. Add dissolved saffron and mussels and cook for 5 minutes, until mussels open. Discard any mussels that do not open. Add marinated shrimp and halibut and cook until fish is tender. Add reserved puréed solids and heat until heated through.

5. **Rouille:** In a mini-chopper, combine mayonnaise, red pepper, garlic and cayenne. Process until smooth. To serve, spread crostini with rouille, place in the bottom of a soup plate and ladle the soup over them.

Cioppino

Tips

To toast fennel seeds: Place seeds in a dry skillet over medium heat, stirring, until fragrant, about 3 minutes. Immediately transfer to a mortar or a spice grinder and grind.

When making cioppino, I like to use Italian San Marzano tomatoes, which are thick and flavorful. If you have access to this excellent product, you can omit the tomato paste.

To prepare shrimp for this recipe, immerse shrimp, in shells, in a large pot of boiling salted water. Cook over high heat until the shells turn pink, about 2 to 3 minutes. Drain and let cool, then peel and devein.

Count 1 tbsp (15 mL) of Easy Rouille as 1 Fat Exchange/Choice.

This zesty stew originated on the San Francisco pier, where it was prepared using whatever was bountiful in the catch that day. The rouille adds flavor and richness. Serve this with a crusty country-style bread, such as ciabatta, and a green salad.

- **Large (minimum 5 quart) slow cooker**

1 tbsp	olive oil	15 mL
2	onions, finely chopped	2
1	bulb fennel, cored and chopped	1
6	cloves garlic, minced	6
4	anchovy fillets, finely chopped	4
1 tsp	cracked black peppercorns	5 mL
½ tsp	fennel seeds, toasted (see Tips, left)	2 mL
1 tbsp	tomato paste (see Tips, left)	15
1	can (28 oz/796 mL) diced tomatoes, including juice	1
1 cup	dry white wine	250 mL
2 cups	bottled clam juice	500 mL
2 cups	water	500 mL
1 lb	skinless firm white fish, such as snapper, cut into bite-size pieces	500 g
8 oz	medium shrimp, cooked, peeled and deveined (see Tips, left)	250 g
8 oz	cooked crabmeat	250 g
1	red bell pepper, diced	1
1	long red chile pepper, diced, optional	1

Easy Rouille (optional)

⅓ cup	mayonnaise	75 mL
2	cloves garlic, puréed	2
1 tbsp	extra virgin olive oil	15 mL
1 tsp	freshly squeezed lemon juice	5 mL
¼ tsp	hot or regular paprika	1 mL

1. In a skillet, heat oil over medium heat for 30 seconds. Add onions and fennel and cook, stirring, until softened, about 3 minutes. Add garlic, anchovies, peppercorns and toasted fennel seeds and cook, stirring, for 1 minute. Stir in tomato paste. Add tomatoes, with juice, and white wine and bring to a boil. Transfer to slow cooker stoneware.

NUTRIENTS PER SERVING	
Calories	152
Fat	3.1 g
Saturates	0.5 g
Polyunsaturates	0.7 g
Monounsaturates	1.3 g
Cholesterol	70 mg
Sodium	612 mg
Carbohydrate	9.3 g
Fiber	2 g
Protein	21.7 g

AMERICA'S EXCHANGES	
2	Vegetable
2½	Very Lean Meat

CANADA'S CHOICES	
½	Carbohydrate
2½	Meat and Alternatives

Make Ahead

This dish can be partially prepared before it is cooked. Complete Step 1. Cover and refrigerate overnight or for up to 2 days. When you're ready to cook, continue with Steps 2 through 4.

2. Add clam juice and water and stir well. Cover and cook on Low for 6 to 8 hours or on High for 3 to 4 hours. Add fish, shrimp, crabmeat, red pepper and chile pepper, if using, and stir well. Cover and cook on High for 20 minutes, until fish flakes easily when pierced with a fork and seafood is heated through.

3. **Easy Rouille (optional):** In a small bowl, combine mayonnaise, garlic, olive oil, lemon juice and paprika. Mix until thoroughly blended.

4. To serve, ladle cioppino into warm bowls and garnish each serving with a dollop of rouille, if using.

Mindful Morsels

Including fennel in your diet is a good way to add variety to what you eat and increase your intake of beneficial antioxidants. Like celery, fennel, a member of the parsley family, is low in calories, but it is more nutritious than celery. One cup (250 mL) of chopped fennel is a source of fiber, folacin and potassium.

Seafood Jambalaya

Like its Spanish relative, paella, jambalaya is an ever-changing mixture depending upon the cook's whim and the available ingredients. This recipe uses Italian sausage instead of the more traditional ham or andouille and produces a medium-spicy result. For more heat, add a hot pepper along with the shrimp. For a more authentic jambalaya, substitute thinly sliced andouille, a Louisiana smoked sausage, for the hot Italian sausage. Since andouille is quite strongly flavored, I suggest using only 8 oz (250 g). Add, along with the shrimp, without browning.

Tips

Large cans of tomatoes come in 28 oz (796 mL) and 35 oz (980 mL) sizes. For convenience, I've called for the 28 oz (796 mL) size in my recipes. If you're using the 35 oz (980 mL) size, drain off 1 cup (250 mL) liquid before adding to the recipe.

To prepare shrimp for this recipe, immerse shrimp, in shells, in a large pot of boiling salted water. Cook over high heat until the shells turn pink, about 2 to 3 minutes. Drain and let cool, then peel and devein.

- **Works best in a large (minimum 5 quart) slow cooker**

1 tbsp	olive oil	15 mL
1 lb	mild Italian sausage, casings removed	500 g
2	onions, finely chopped	2
2	stalks celery, cut into ¼-inch (0.5 cm) dice	2
4	cloves garlic, finely chopped	4
½ tsp	salt	2 mL
1 tsp	dried thyme leaves	5 mL
1 tsp	dried oregano leaves	5 mL
½ tsp	cracked black peppercorns	2 mL
1	bay leaf	1
2 cups	lower-salt chicken broth	500 mL
1	can (28 oz/796 mL) diced tomatoes, including juice (see Tips, left)	1
8 oz	boneless skinless chicken breasts or thighs, cut into 1-inch (2.5 cm) cubes	250 g
2 cups	long-grain rice, preferably parboiled	500 mL
1 lb	medium shrimp, cooked, peeled and deveined (see Tips, left)	500 g
2 tbsp	Worcestershire sauce	25 mL
1	hot banana pepper or long red or green chile, finely chopped, optional	1

1. In a skillet, heat oil over medium-high heat for 30 seconds. Add sausage and cook, breaking up with a spoon, until no longer pink, about 10 minutes. Using a slotted spoon, transfer to slow cooker stoneware. Drain all but 1 tbsp (15 mL) fat from pan.

NUTRIENTS PER SERVING	
Calories	280
Fat	8.4 g
Saturates	2.6 g
Polyunsaturates	1.2 g
Monounsaturates	4.0 g
Cholesterol	86 mg
Sodium	623 mg
Carbohydrate	30.7 g
Fiber	1.6 g
Protein	19.2 g

AMERICA'S EXCHANGES	
2	Starch
2	Lean Meat

CANADA'S CHOICES	
2	Carbohydrate
2	Meat and Alternatives

Make Ahead

This dish can be partially prepared before it is cooked. Complete Steps 1 and 2. Cover and refrigerate sausage and vegetable mixtures separately for up to 2 days. Cook, peel and devein shrimp and refrigerate overnight. The next day, combine sausage and vegetables in slow cooker stoneware and continue with the recipe.

2. Reduce heat to medium. Add onions and celery and cook, stirring, until softened, about 5 minutes. Add garlic, salt, thyme, oregano and peppercorns and cook, stirring, for 1 minute. Add bay leaf, broth and tomatoes with juice and bring to a boil. Transfer to slow cooker.

3. Add chicken and rice and stir well. Place two clean tea towels, each folded in half (so you will have four layers), across the top of the stoneware to absorb moisture. Cover and cook on Low for 6 to 8 hours or on High for 3 to 4 hours. Stir in shrimp, Worcestershire sauce and hot pepper, if using. Cover and cook on High for 20 to 30 minutes, or until shrimp are heated through. Discard bay leaf and serve.

Mindful Morsels

To increase the nutritional value of this dish, substitute long-grain brown rice for the white. Brown rice contains much more fiber than white rice — $\frac{1}{2}$ cup (125 mL) of white rice contains 0.3 g of dietary fiber, while you'll get 1.5 g from the same quantity of brown.

Onion-Braised Shrimp

This is a great dish for a buffet, an Indian-style meal with numerous small plates or a light dinner. The substantial quantity of onions, which are cooked until they begin to caramelize and release their sugars, produces a dish that is pleasantly sweet. I like to serve this over long-grain brown rice.

Tips

The quantity of pepper in the recipe produces a mildly spicy result, but the sweetness of the onions can balance more heat, if desired. Heat seekers can add an extra half of a fresh chile, finely chopped, or more cayenne pepper. You can add up to ½ tsp (2 mL) cayenne pepper in addition to the fresh red chile. Just be sure to dissolve the powdered pepper in the lemon juice before adding to the slow cooker.

If your supermarket has 19-oz (540 mL) cans of diced tomatoes, by all means substitute that size in this recipe.

If you don't have a fresh chile, use ½ tsp (2 mL) cayenne pepper instead. Dissolve it in the lemon juice before adding to the slow cooker.

Make Ahead

This dish can be partially prepared before it is cooked. Complete Steps 1 and 2. Cover and refrigerate overnight or for up to 2 days. When you're ready to cook, continue with Step 3.

- **Works in slow cookers from 3½ to 6 quarts**

1 tsp	coriander seeds	5 mL
1 tbsp	olive oil	15 mL
4	onions, finely chopped	4
2	cloves garlic, minced	2
1 tbsp	minced gingerroot	15 mL
1 tsp	turmeric	5 mL
1 tsp	salt	5 mL
½ tsp	cracked black peppercorns	2 mL
1	can (14 oz/398 mL) diced tomatoes, including juice (see Tips, left)	1
1	long red chile pepper, seeded and finely chopped (see Tips, left)	1
1 tbsp	freshly squeezed lemon juice	15 mL
1 lb	medium shrimp, cooked, peeled and deveined (see Tips, page 154)	500 g
½ cup	low-fat plain yogurt	125 mL
2 tbsp	finely chopped cilantro leaves	25 mL

1. In a dry skillet over medium heat, toast coriander seeds, stirring, until fragrant, about 3 minutes. Immediately transfer to a mortar or a spice grinder and grind. Set aside.

2. In same skillet, heat oil over medium heat for 30 seconds. Add onions and cook, stirring, until they turn golden and just begin to brown, about 7 minutes. Add garlic, gingerroot, turmeric, salt, peppercorns and reserved coriander and cook, stirring, for 1 minute. Add tomatoes with juice and stir well. Transfer to slow cooker stoneware.

3. Cover and cook on Low for 6 hours or on High for 3 hours, until mixture is hot and bubbly. Stir in chile pepper and lemon juice. Add shrimp and stir well. Cover and cook on High for 20 minutes, until shrimp are heated through. Stir in yogurt. Garnish with cilantro and serve.

NUTRIENTS PER SERVING	
Calories	163
Fat	4.5 g
Saturates	1.0 g
Polyunsaturates	0.8 g
Monounsaturates	2.1 g
Cholesterol	117 mg
Sodium	319 mg
Carbohydrate	12.9 g
Fiber	2.0 g
Protein	18.1 g

AMERICA'S EXCHANGES	
2½	Vegetable
2	Lean Meat

CANADA'S CHOICES	
½	Carbohydrate
2	Meat and Alternatives

Tips

Coconut oil is traditionally used in tropical cuisines. It has a much higher proportion of saturated fatty acids in relation to the unsaturated kind, which makes it more chemically stable and much less prone to rancidity in hot conditions, an important consideration before the advent of refrigeration. (See also page 68.)

If you are adding the almond garnish, try to find slivered almonds with the skin on. They add color and nutrients to the dish.

Make Ahead

This dish can be partially prepared before it is cooked. Complete Step 1. Cover and refrigerate overnight or for up to 2 days. When you're ready to cook, continue with Steps 2 and 3.

Sweet Potato Coconut Curry with Shrimp

I love the combination of sweet and spicy flavors in this luscious dish. Serve this over brown basmati rice and add a platter of steamed spinach lightly sprinkled with toasted sesame seeds to complete the meal.

- **Works in slow cookers from 3½ to 6 quarts**

1 tbsp	olive or extra virgin coconut oil	15 mL
2	onions, finely chopped	2
4	cloves garlic, minced	4
1 tbsp	minced gingerroot	15 mL
1 cup	lower-salt vegetable broth	250 mL
2	sweet potatoes, peeled and cut into 1-inch (2.5 cm) cubes	2
2 tsp	Thai green curry paste	10 mL
1 tbsp	freshly squeezed lime juice	15
½ cup	coconut milk	125 mL
1 lb	medium shrimp, cooked, peeled and deveined (see Tips, page 154)	500 g
¼ cup	toasted slivered almonds, optional (see Tips, left)	50 mL
¼ cup	finely chopped cilantro leaves	50 mL

1. In a skillet, heat oil over medium heat for 30 seconds. Add onions and cook, stirring, until softened, about 3 minutes. Add garlic and gingerroot and cook, stirring, for 1 minute. Add broth. Transfer to slow cooker stoneware.

2. Add sweet potatoes and stir well. Cover and cook on Low for 6 to 8 hours or on High for 3 to 4 hours, until sweet potatoes are tender.

3. In a small bowl, combine curry paste and lime juice. Add to slow cooker stoneware and stir well. Stir in coconut milk and shrimp. Cover and cook on High for 20 minutes, until shrimp are hot. Transfer to a serving dish. Garnish with almonds, if using, and cilantro and serve.

NUTRIENTS PER SERVING	
Calories	232
Fat	8.2 g
Saturates	4.2 g
Polyunsaturates	0.9 g
Monounsaturates	2.5 g
Cholesterol	147 mg
Sodium	355 mg
Carbohydrate	21.8 g
Fiber	1.9 g
Protein	18.0 g

AMERICA'S EXCHANGES	
1	Starch
1	Vegetable
2	Very Lean Meat
1	Fat

CANADA'S CHOICES	
1	Carbohydrate
2	Meat and Alternatives
1	Extra

Tips

Large cans of tomatoes come in 28 oz (796 mL) and 35 oz (980 mL) sizes. For convenience, I've called for the 28 oz (796 mL) size in my recipes.

To prepare shrimp for this recipe, immerse shrimp, in shells, in a large pot of boiling salted water. Cook over high heat until the shells turn pink, about 2 to 3 minutes. Drain and let cool, then peel and devein.

Chile nomenclature can be confusing. Long red or green chiles are usually used in Indian cooking and can be found in Asian markets. They are sometimes called cayenne or serrano chiles, not to be confused with Mexican serrano chiles, which are different.

Make Ahead

This dish can be partially prepared, in stages, before it is cooked. Complete Step 1. Cover and refrigerate mixture for up to 2 days. Chop parsley, zest lemon and slice green pepper. Cover and refrigerate overnight. Cook shrimp. Peel and devein and refrigerate overnight. The next day, continue with the recipe.

NUTRIENTS PER SERVING	
Calories	177
Fat	4.9 g
Saturates	0.8 g
Polyunsaturates	0.9 g
Monounsaturates	2.7 g
Cholesterol	169 mg
Sodium	694 mg
Carbohydrate	13.6 g
Fiber	2.9 g
Protein	20.9 g

Shrimp Creole

This classic Louisiana dish needs only fluffy rice or hot crusty bread and a green salad to make a delicious meal. For a special treat, add crisp white wine.

- **Works in slow cookers from 3½ to 6 quarts**

1 tbsp	olive oil	15 mL
1	onion, finely chopped	1
4	stalks celery, cut into ¼-inch (0.5 cm) dice	4
2	cloves garlic, minced	2
1 tsp	dried oregano leaves	5 mL
½ tsp	dried thyme leaves	2 mL
¼ tsp	salt	1 mL
½ tsp	cracked black peppercorns	2 mL
1	can (28 oz/796 mL) diced tomatoes, drained (see Tips, left)	1
¼ cup	bottled clam juice	50 mL
¼ cup	water	50 mL
¼ cup	finely chopped parsley	50 mL
	Grated zest of 1 lemon	
1 tbsp	Worcestershire sauce	15 mL
1 lb	medium shrimp, cooked, peeled and deveined (see Tips, left)	500 g
1	green bell pepper, thinly sliced	1
½ to 1	long red or green chile pepper, finely chopped (see Tips, left)	½ to 1
	Hot cooked rice	

1. In a skillet, heat oil over medium heat for 30 seconds. Add onion and celery and cook, stirring, until softened, about 5 minutes. Add garlic, oregano, thyme, salt and peppercorns and cook, stirring, for 1 minute. Add tomatoes, clam juice and water and bring to a boil. Transfer to slow cooker stoneware.

2. Cover and cook on Low for 6 to 8 hours or on High for 3 to 4 hours, until hot and bubbly. Add parsley, lemon zest and Worcestershire sauce and stir. Add shrimp, green pepper and chile pepper and stir thoroughly. Cover and cook on High for 20 minutes, or until peppers are soft and shrimp are heated through. Serve over hot rice.

AMERICA'S EXCHANGES	
2½	Vegetable
2½	Very Lean Meat
½	Fat

CANADA'S CHOICES	
½	Carbohydrate
2½	Meat and Alternatives

Poultry

(1 piece of chicken with rice per serving)

Tip

Mixtures of wild and several varieties of brown rice now come in packages. Use plain brown rice instead, or you can make your own mixture by combining ¾ cup (175 mL) of each.

Sage and Onion Chicken with Cranberry Rice

Simple but tasty, this dish has all the flavors of the Christmas turkey without the work. Add a tossed green salad or some marinated roasted red peppers to complete the meal.

- **Works best in a large (minimum 5 quart) slow cooker**
- **Lightly greased slow cooker stoneware**

1 tbsp	olive oil	15 mL
2	onions, finely chopped	2
4	cloves garlic, minced	4
1½ tsp	dried sage leaves	7 mL
½ tsp	cracked black peppercorns	2 mL
½ tsp	salt	2 mL
1 lb	mushrooms, sliced	500 g
1½ cups	brown and wild rice mixture, rinsed (see Tip, left)	375 mL
1 cup	dried cranberries	250 mL
3 cups	lower-salt chicken broth	750 mL
	Grated zest and juice of 1 orange	
3 lbs	skinless bone-in chicken thighs (about 12 thighs)	1.5 kg

Topping

1 tbsp	butter	15 mL
1 tbsp	olive oil	15 mL
1 cup	fresh whole wheat bread crumbs	250 mL
2 tbsp	toasted sliced almonds	25 mL

1. In a skillet, heat oil over medium heat for 30 seconds. Add onions and cook, stirring, until softened, about 3 minutes. Add garlic, sage, peppercorns and salt and cook, stirring, for 1 minute. Add mushrooms and stir to coat. Add rice and stir to coat. Stir in cranberries. Add broth, orange zest and juice and bring to a boil. (You should have 4 cups/ 1 L of liquid in total. Squeeze the orange juice into a 1 cup/250 mL measure and add broth to make up the 1 cup/250 mL, if necessary.)

2. Spoon half the rice mixture evenly over bottom of prepared slow cooker stoneware. Arrange chicken pieces evenly over top. Cover with remaining rice mixture.

NUTRIENTS PER SERVING	
Calories	275
Fat	8.7 g
Saturates	2.2 g
Polyunsaturates	1.6 g
Monounsaturates	4.1 g
Cholesterol	55 mg
Sodium	301 mg
Carbohydrate	31.9 g
Fiber	3.5 g
Protein	18.2 g

AMERICA'S EXCHANGES	
2	Starch
2	Lean Meat

CANADA'S CHOICES	
2	Carbohydrate
2	Meat and Alternatives

Make Ahead

This dish can be partially prepared before it is cooked. Complete Step 1. Cover and refrigerate overnight. The next morning, continue with the recipe.

3. Place two clean tea towels, each folded in half (so you will have four layers), over top of stoneware to absorb moisture. Cover and cook on Low for 6 hours or on High for 3 hours, until juices run clear when chicken is pierced with a fork.

4. **Topping:** In a skillet, heat butter and oil over medium heat. Add bread crumbs and toss until evenly coated. Cook, stirring, until golden, about 5 minutes. Stir in almonds. Spoon evenly over cooked rice and serve immediately.

Mindful Morsels

Cranberries (along with cherries, blueberries and other red, purple and blue fruits) are particularly good sources of anthocyanins and other antioxidants that protect all cells in the body.

Make Ahead

This recipe can be partially prepared before it is cooked. Complete Step 1. Cover and refrigerate for up to 2 days. When you're ready to cook, continue with the recipe.

Balsamic Braised Chicken with Olives

Here's a tasty Mediterranean-inspired dish that is simple yet elegant. Serve this over creamy Basic Polenta (see recipe, page 229) or hot whole grain couscous for a delectable meal.

- **Works best in a large (minimum 5 quart) slow cooker**

1 tbsp	olive oil	15 mL
2	onions, finely chopped	2
4	cloves garlic, minced	4
½ tsp	salt	2 mL
½ tsp	cracked black peppercorns	2 mL
½ tsp	dried thyme leaves	2 mL
2 cups	chopped peeled tomatoes, including juice, if canned	500 mL
½ cup	lower-salt chicken broth	125 mL
2 tbsp	balsamic vinegar	25 mL
3 lbs	skinless bone-in chicken thighs (about 12 thighs)	1.5 kg
2 tbsp	chopped pitted black olives	25 mL
2 tbsp	drained capers	25 mL

1. In a skillet, heat oil over medium heat for 30 seconds. Add onions and cook, stirring, until softened, about 3 minutes. Add garlic, salt, peppercorns and thyme and cook, stirring, for 1 minute. Add tomatoes with juice, broth and balsamic vinegar and bring to a boil.

2. Arrange chicken over bottom of slow cooker stoneware and cover with vegetable mixture. Cover and cook on Low for 6 hours or on High for 3 hours, until juices run clear when chicken is pierced with a fork. Add olives and capers and stir well. Serve immediately.

NUTRIENTS PER SERVING	
Calories	123
Fat	5.3 g
Saturates	1.3 g
Polyunsaturates	1.1 g
Monounsaturates	2.4 g
Cholesterol	53 mg
Sodium	226 mg
Carbohydrate	3.9 g
Fiber	0.8 g
Protein	14.5 g

AMERICA'S EXCHANGES	
2	Lean Meat

CANADA'S CHOICES	
2	Meat and Alternatives

MAKES 12 SERVINGS
(1 piece of chicken with barley per serving)

Tip

Use whole, pot or pearl barley in this recipe.

Make Ahead

This recipe can be partially prepared before it is cooked. Complete Step 1. Cover and refrigerate for up to 2 days. When you're ready to cook, continue with the recipe.

Chicken and Barley

I love the simple but appetizing combination of flavors in this delicious dish. Although we usually eat this as a family dinner, all it takes is a dressed-up salad — try a combination of Boston lettuce, mesclun greens, red onion and avocado in a balsamic vinaigrette — crusty rolls and some crisp white wine to make it perfect for guests.

- **Works best in a large (minimum 5 quart) slow cooker**

1 tbsp	olive oil	15 mL
2	onions, chopped	2
4	stalks celery, diced	4
4	cloves garlic, minced	4
1 tsp	salt	5 mL
½ tsp	cracked black peppercorns	2 mL
½ tsp	dried thyme leaves	2 mL
1 cup	barley, rinsed (see Tip, left)	250 mL
1	can (28 oz/796 mL) diced tomatoes, including juice	1
1 cup	dry white wine or lower-salt chicken broth	250 mL
3 lbs	skinless bone-in chicken thighs (about 12 thighs)	1.5 kg
2	red bell peppers, chopped	2
	Finely chopped dill	

1. In a skillet, heat oil over medium heat for 30 seconds. Add onions and celery and cook, stirring, until softened, about 5 minutes. Add garlic, salt, peppercorns and thyme and cook, stirring, for 1 minute. Add barley and stir until coated. Add tomatoes, with juice, and wine and bring to a boil.

2. Arrange chicken over bottom of slow cooker stoneware and cover with vegetable mixture. Cover and cook on Low for 6 hours or on High for 3 hours, until juices run clear when chicken is pierced with a fork. Add peppers and cook on High for 15 minutes, until softened. Transfer mixture to a deep platter and garnish liberally with dill. Serve piping hot.

NUTRIENTS PER SERVING	
Calories	192
Fat	5.5 g
Saturates	1.3 g
Polyunsaturates	1.2 g
Monounsaturates	2.4 g
Cholesterol	53 mg
Sodium	368 mg
Carbohydrate	19.9 g
Fiber	2.4 g
Protein	16.1 g

AMERICA'S EXCHANGES	
1	Starch
1	Vegetable
1½	Lean Meat

CANADA'S CHOICES	
1	Carbohydrate
2	Meat and Alternatives

Tip

Because the chicken only cooks for 6 hours on Low, the potatoes will be a bit firm unless they are blanched (see Step 1) before they are added to the stew.

Make Ahead

This dish can be partially prepared before it is cooked. Complete Steps 1 and 2. Cover and refrigerate overnight. The next morning, continue with the recipe.

Classic Chicken Stew

I have a real soft spot for this creamy stew, which reminds me of chicken pot pie without the crust. I obtain a similar effect by serving it over crostini placed in the bottom of a soup plate. Add a tossed green salad for a complete and delicious meal.

• **Works best in a large (minimum 5 quart) slow cooker**

1	potato, peeled and diced	1
1 tbsp	olive oil	15 mL
2	onions, finely chopped	2
4	stalks celery, diced	4
2	carrots, peeled and diced	2
½ tsp	dried thyme leaves or 3 whole sprigs of fresh thyme	2 mL
1	bay leaf	1
¼ cup	all-purpose flour	50 mL
1½ cups	lower-salt chicken broth	375 mL
½ cup	dry white wine or lower-salt chicken broth	125 mL
	Freshly ground black pepper	
3 lbs	skinless bone-in chicken thighs (about 12 thighs)	1.5 kg
1 cup	green peas, thawed if frozen	250 mL

1. In a saucepan, combine potato and cold water to cover. Bring to a boil and cook for 2 minutes. Remove from heat. Cover and set aside.

2. In a skillet, heat oil over medium heat for 30 seconds. Add onions, celery and carrots and cook, stirring, until carrots are softened, about 7 minutes. Add thyme, bay leaf and flour and cook, stirring, for 1 minute. Add broth and white wine and cook, stirring, until mixture comes to a boil and thickens, about 4 minutes. Drain reserved potato and add to mixture. Season to taste with pepper.

3. Arrange chicken over bottom of slow cooker stoneware and cover with vegetable mixture. Cover and cook on Low for 6 hours or on High for 3 hours, until juices run clear when chicken is pierced with a fork. Add peas and stir well. Cover and cook on High for 20 minutes, until peas are tender and mixture is hot and bubbly.

NUTRIENTS PER SERVING	
Calories	145
Fat	5.2 g
Saturates	1.3 g
Polyunsaturates	1.0 g
Monounsaturates	2.3 g
Cholesterol	53 mg
Sodium	139 mg
Carbohydrate	8.4 g
Fiber	1.5 g
Protein	15.6 g

AMERICA'S EXCHANGES	
1½	Vegetable
2	Lean Meat

CANADA'S CHOICES	
½	Carbohydrate
2	Meat and Alternatives

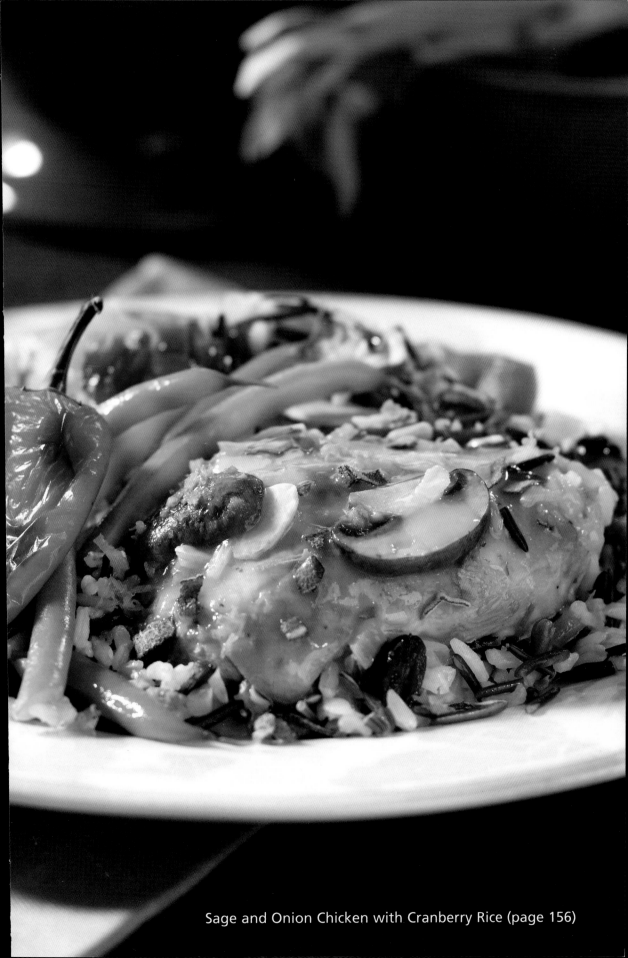

Sage and Onion Chicken with Cranberry Rice (page 156)

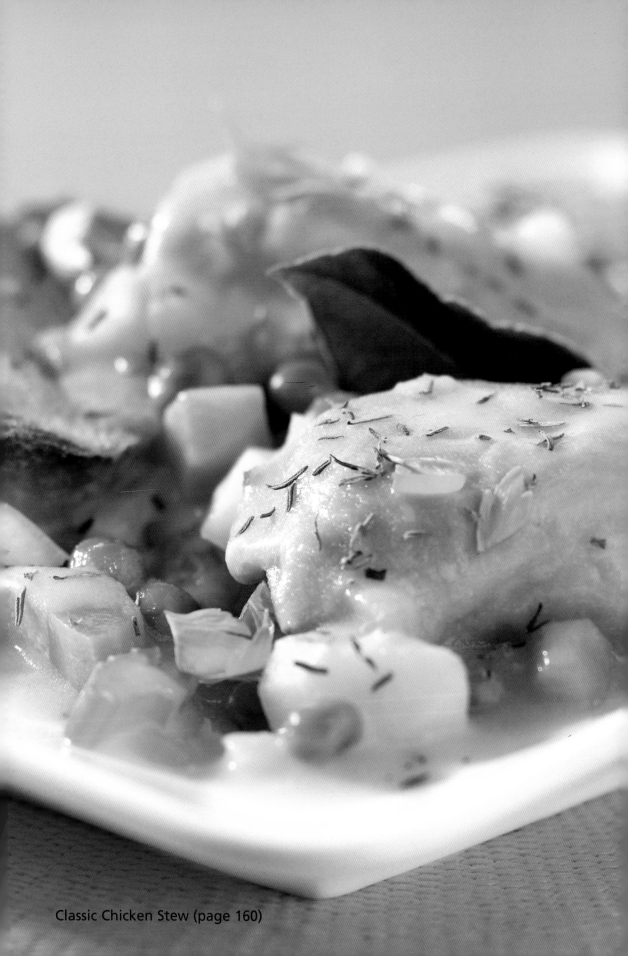

Classic Chicken Stew (page 160)

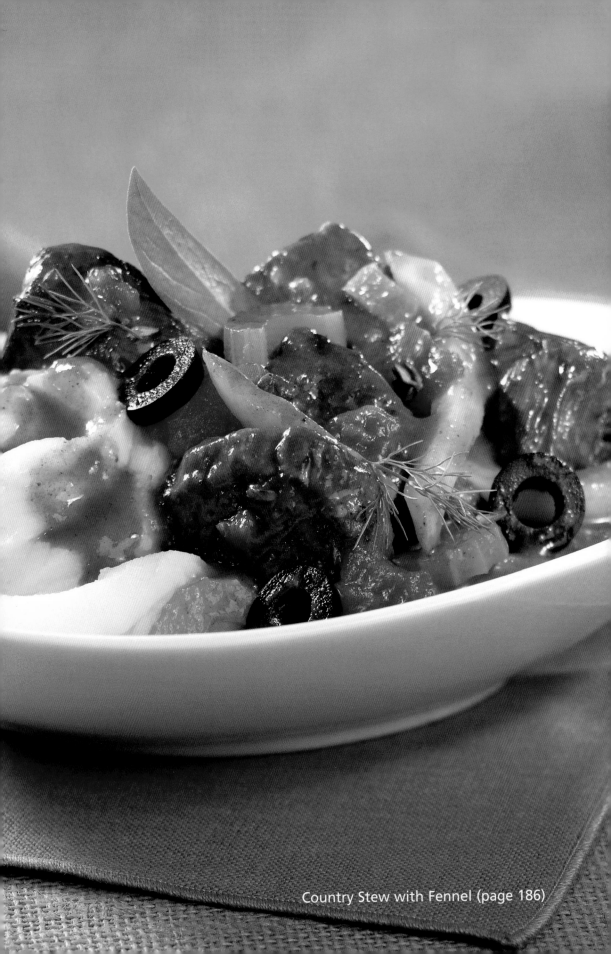

Country Stew with Fennel (page 186)

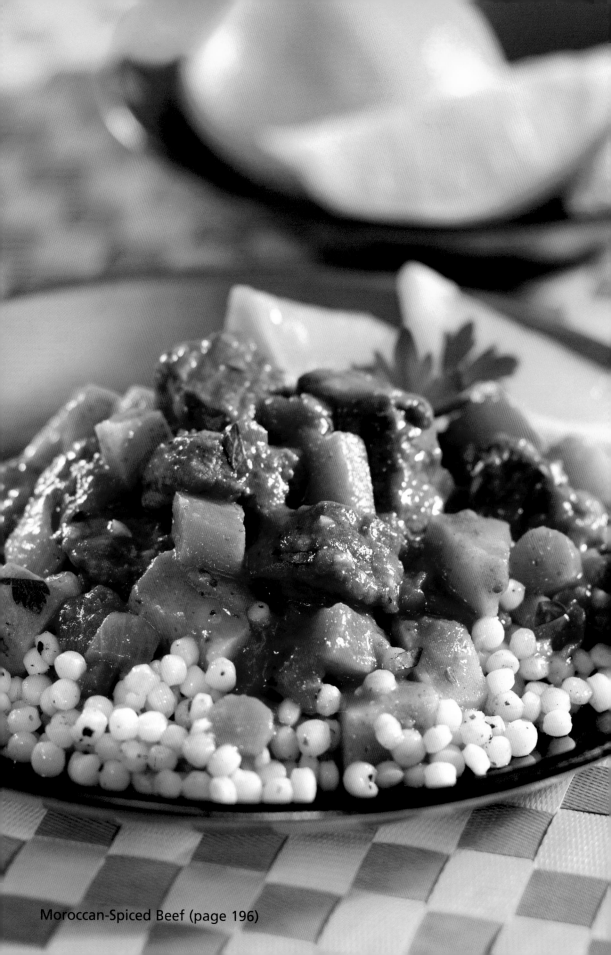
Moroccan-Spiced Beef (page 196)

(1 piece of chicken with vegetables per serving)

Tip

I like to use Italian San Marzano tomatoes when making this recipe because they have more flavor than domestic varieties. If you can't find them, add 1 tbsp (15 mL) tomato paste along with the tomatoes.

Make Ahead

This dish can be partially prepared before it is cooked. Complete Step 1. Cover and refrigerate overnight or for up to 2 days. When you're ready to cook, continue with Steps 2 and 3.

Chicken Cacciatore with Broccoli

This dish is a classic because it's so tasty. The addition of broccoli to the traditional ingredients adds flavor as well as nutrients. Serve this over hot polenta or whole grain pasta for a delicious meal.

- **Large (minimum 5 quart) slow cooker**

2 tbsp	olive oil, divided	25 mL
2	onions, finely chopped	2
4	cloves garlic, minced	4
1 tsp	dried oregano leaves, crumbled	5 mL
½ tsp	salt	2 mL
½ tsp	cracked black peppercorns	2 mL
8 oz	cremini mushrooms, trimmed and sliced	250 g
1 cup	dry white wine or lower-salt chicken broth	250 mL
1	can (28 oz/796 mL) diced tomatoes, including juice (see Tip, left)	1
3 lbs	skinless bone-in chicken thighs (about 12 thighs)	1.5 kg
2	dried red chile peppers, optional	2
1	green bell pepper, diced	1
4 cups	broccoli florets, blanched	1 L

1. In a skillet, heat 1 tbsp (15 mL) of the olive oil over medium heat for 30 seconds. Add onions and cook, stirring, until softened, about 3 minutes. Add garlic, oregano, salt and peppercorns and cook, stirring, for 1 minute. Add mushrooms and toss to coat. Add white wine and tomatoes with juice and bring to a boil.

2. Arrange chicken over bottom of slow cooker stoneware. Cover with sauce. Cover and cook on Low for 6 hours or on High for 3 hours, until juices run clear when chicken is pierced with a fork. Using a slotted spoon, transfer chicken to a heatproof serving dish and keep warm in oven.

3. In a skillet, heat remaining 1 tbsp (15 mL) of the oil over medium heat for 30 seconds. Add chile peppers, if using, and cook, stirring, for 1 minute. Add bell pepper and cook, stirring, until softened, about 3 minutes. Add tomato sauce from slow cooker stoneware and bring to a boil. Reduce heat and simmer until slightly reduced and thickened, about 10 minutes. Add broccoli and cook until heated through. Combine with chicken and serve.

NUTRIENTS PER SERVING	
Calories	159
Fat	6.7 g
Saturates	1.4 g
Polyunsaturates	1.4 g
Monounsaturates	1.8 g
Cholesterol	69 mg
Sodium	273 mg
Carbohydrate	7.3 g
Fiber	1.8 g
Protein	17.8 g

AMERICA'S EXCHANGES	
1½	Vegetable
2½	Lean Meat

CANADA'S CHOICES	
2	Meat and Alternatives
1	Extra

MAKES 8 SERVINGS
(1 piece of chicken with
beans per serving)

Tip

If you're using small cremini mushrooms (my preference in this recipe), just remove the stems and use them whole. Cut larger ones in half or quarters, depending on the size. If using portobello mushrooms, remove the stems and gills and cut each cap into 6 equal wedges.

Make Ahead

This dish can be partially prepared before it is cooked. Complete Step 1. Cover and refrigerate bean mixture for up to 2 days. When you're ready to cook, continue with Steps 2 and 3.

Chicken Cassoulet

This hearty one-dish meal is always a hit — I particularly like the dill finish, which adds an intriguing hint of flavor. I like to serve this with whole grain bread to soak up the luscious sauce. A salad of shredded carrots makes a nice accompaniment.

- **Large (minimum 6 quart) slow cooker**

1 tbsp	olive oil	15 mL
2	onions, finely chopped	2
8	carrots, peeled and sliced	8
4	stalks celery, sliced	4
4	cloves garlic, minced	4
2 tsp	herbes de Provence	10 mL
½ tsp	salt	2 mL
1 tsp	cracked black peppercorns	5 mL
1	can (28 oz/796 mL) diced tomatoes, including juice	1
1 cup	lower-salt chicken or vegetable broth	250 mL
2	cans (each 14 oz/398 mL) white beans, rinsed and drained, or 2 cups (500 mL) dried white beans, soaked, cooked and drained (see Basic Beans, page 231)	2
2	bay leaves	2
2 lbs	skinless bone-in chicken thighs (about 8 thighs)	1 kg
1 lb	cremini or portobello mushrooms (see Tip, left)	500 g
½ cup	finely chopped dill	125 mL

1. In a large skillet, heat oil over medium heat for 30 seconds. Add onions, carrots and celery and cook, stirring, until carrots are softened, about 7 minutes. Add garlic, herbes de Provence, salt and peppercorns and cook, stirring, for 1 minute. Add tomatoes with juice, broth, beans and bay leaves and bring to a boil. Remove from heat.

2. Spoon half of the bean mixture into slow cooker stoneware. Lay chicken evenly over top. Arrange mushrooms evenly over chicken. Spoon remainder of sauce over mushrooms.

3. Cover and cook on Low for 6 hours or on High for 3 hours, until juices run clear when chicken is pierced with a fork. Stir in dill. Cover and cook on High for 15 minutes, until flavors meld.

NUTRIENTS PER SERVING	
Calories	281
Fat	6.8 g
Saturates	1.4 g
Polyunsaturates	2.6 g
Monounsaturates	1.5 g
Cholesterol	69 mg
Sodium	762 mg
Carbohydrate	32.7 g
Fiber	10.3 g
Protein	24.4 g

AMERICA'S EXCHANGES	
2	Starch
2½	Extra-lean Meat
½	Fat

CANADA'S CHOICES	
1½	Carbohydrate
3	Meat and Alternatives

MAKES 12 SERVINGS
(1 piece of chicken with
vegetables per serving)

Tips

If you prefer, substitute an equal
amount of lower-salt chicken
broth for the wine.

If your supermarket carries
19-oz (540 mL) cans of diced
tomatoes, by all means
substitute for the 14 oz (398 mL)
called for in the recipe.

Make Ahead

This recipe can be partially
prepared before it is cooked.
Complete Step 1. Cover and
refrigerate overnight or for up to
2 days. When you're ready to
cook, continue with Step 2.

French Basil Chicken

*I call this French Basil Chicken to distinguish it from the well-
known dish Thai basil chicken, which is also a staple at our house.
This version combines chicken with the complementary flavors of
tomato, artichoke and sweet red pepper. A healthy quantity of finely
chopped fresh basil leaves is stirred in at the end.*

- **Works in slow cookers from 3½ to 6 quarts**

1 tbsp	olive oil	15 mL
2	onions, finely chopped	2
4	cloves garlic, minced	4
1 tsp	herbes de Provence	5 mL
½ tsp	salt	2 mL
½ tsp	cracked black peppercorns	2 mL
1 tbsp	all-purpose flour	15 mL
½ cup	dry white wine (see Tips, left)	125 mL
1 cup	lower-salt chicken broth	250 mL
1	can (14 oz/398 mL) diced tomatoes, including juice (see Tips, left)	1
1	can (14 oz/398 mL) artichoke hearts, drained, rinsed and quartered	1
3 lbs	skinless bone-in chicken thighs (about 12 thighs)	1.5 kg
2 cups	diced red bell pepper	500 mL
½ cup	finely chopped fresh basil leaves	125 mL

1. In a skillet, heat oil over medium heat for 30 seconds. Add
   onions and cook, stirring, until softened, about 3 minutes.
   Add garlic, herbes de Provence, salt and peppercorns and
   cook, stirring, for 1 minute. Add flour and cook, stirring,
   for 1 minute. Add wine and cook, stirring, for 1 minute.
   Add broth and tomatoes with juice and bring to a boil.
   Stir in artichoke hearts and remove from heat.

2. Arrange chicken pieces evenly over the bottom of slow
   cooker stoneware and cover with tomato mixture. Cover
   and cook on Low for 6 hours or on High for 3 hours, until
   juices run clear when chicken is pierced with a fork. Stir
   in red pepper and basil. Cover and cook on High for
   30 minutes, or until pepper is tender.

NUTRIENTS PER SERVING	
Calories	153
Fat	5.5 g
Saturates	1.3 g
Polyunsaturates	1.2 g
Monounsaturates	2.1 g
Cholesterol	69 mg
Sodium	339 mg
Carbohydrate	8.3 g
Fiber	2.3 g
Protein	17.7 g

AMERICA'S EXCHANGES	
1½	Vegetable
2	Lean Meat

CANADA'S CHOICES	
½	Carbohydrate
2	Meat and Alternatives

Tip

For optimum results, make an effort to find fresh sage, which is often available in the produce section of well-stocked supermarkets or specialty stores. If you can't locate it, dried sage is an acceptable substitute in this recipe.

Make Ahead

This dish can be partially prepared before it is cooked. Complete Step 3, heating 1 tbsp (15 mL) of the oil in pan before softening onions. Cover and refrigerate overnight. The next morning, continue with the recipe.

Tuscan Chicken with Sage

This simple yet delicious chicken gets its distinctive, slightly peppery flavor from the addition of fresh sage, which has a pleasantly pungent flavor. In many ways, it's an Italian variation of coq au vin. Serve with a basic risotto, a robust green vegetable, such as broccoli or rapini, and hot crusty bread to soak up the sauce.

• **Works best in a large (minimum 5 quart) slow cooker**

3 lbs	skinless bone-in chicken thighs (about 12 thighs)	1.5 kg
½ cup	all-purpose flour	125 mL
2 tbsp	olive oil	25 mL
2	onions, finely chopped	2
2	cloves garlic, minced	2
½ cup	fresh sage leaves or 1 tsp (5 mL) dried sage (see Tip, left)	125 mL
1 tsp	salt	5 mL
½ tsp	cracked black peppercorns	2 mL
2 cups	dry robust red wine, such as Chianti	500 mL

1. On a plate, coat chicken on all sides with flour, shaking off the excess. Discard excess flour.

2. In a skillet, heat oil over medium-high heat for 30 seconds. Add chicken, in batches, and brown on all sides. Transfer to slow cooker stoneware.

3. Reduce heat to medium. Add onions to pan, adding additional oil, if needed. Cook, stirring, until softened, about 3 minutes. Add garlic, sage, salt and peppercorns and cook, stirring, for 1 minute. Pour in wine, bring to boil and cook, stirring, for 5 minutes, until sauce is reduced by one-third.

4. Pour mixture over chicken. Cover and cook on Low for 5 hours or on High for 2½ hours, until juices run clear when chicken is pierced with a fork. Serve immediately.

NUTRIENTS PER SERVING	
Calories	189
Fat	8.0 g
Saturates	1.9 g
Polyunsaturates	1.5 g
Monounsaturates	3.8 g
Cholesterol	76 mg
Sodium	268 mg
Carbohydrate	6.6 g
Fiber	0.4 g
Protein	21.0 g

AMERICA'S EXCHANGES	
1½	Vegetable
3	Lean Meat

CANADA'S CHOICES	
½	Carbohydrate
3	Meat and Alternatives

MAKES 12 SERVINGS
(1 piece of chicken with
sauce per serving)

Tip

Count ½ cup (125 mL) cooked rice as a Starch Exchange/Carbohydrate Choice.

Make Ahead

This recipe can be partially prepared before it is cooked. Complete Step 1. Cover and refrigerate for up to 2 days. When you're ready to cook, continue with the recipe.

NUTRIENTS PER SERVING	
Calories	161
Fat	9.5 g
Saturates	5.1 g
Polyunsaturates	1.1 g
Monounsaturates	2.5 g
Cholesterol	53 mg
Sodium	99 mg
Carbohydrate	4.1 g
Fiber	0.6 g
Protein	15.0 g

The Captain's Curry

This style of curry, made with a creamed curry sauce, was popular in the great American seaports during the 19th century. It gets its name from sea captains involved in the spice trade, who brought their wares to cities such as Charleston. Today, we associate coconut milk with our current interest in Asian foods. But citizens of the old South were quite familiar with this ingredient, which they made themselves using fresh coconuts from the West Indies.

- **Works best in a large (minimum 5 quart) slow cooker**

1 tbsp	olive oil	15 mL
2	onions, finely chopped	2
2	stalks celery, thinly sliced	2
2	cloves garlic, minced	2
½ tsp	ground allspice	2 mL
½ tsp	freshly grated nutmeg	2 mL
1	piece (3 inches/7.5 cm) cinnamon stick	1
1	bay leaf	1
2 tbsp	all-purpose flour	25 mL
1 cup	lower-salt chicken broth	250 mL
3 lbs	skinless bone-in chicken thighs (about 12 thighs)	1.5 kg
1 cup	coconut milk, divided	250 mL
1 tbsp	curry powder	15 mL
½ tsp	cayenne pepper	2 mL
	Hot white rice	

1. In a skillet, heat oil over medium heat for 30 seconds. Add onions and celery and cook, stirring, until celery is softened, about 5 minutes. Add garlic, allspice, nutmeg, cinnamon stick and bay leaf and cook, stirring, for 1 minute. Sprinkle flour over mixture and cook, stirring, for 1 minute. Add broth. Bring to a boil and cook, stirring, until thickened.

2. Arrange chicken over bottom of slow cooker stoneware and cover with vegetable mixture. Cover and cook on Low for 6 hours or on High for 3 hours, until juices run clear when chicken is pierced with a fork.

3. In a small bowl, combine ¼ cup (50 mL) of the coconut milk with curry powder and cayenne. Mix well. Add to stoneware. Stir in remaining coconut milk and cook on High for 30 minutes, until flavors meld. Discard cinnamon stick and bay leaf. Serve over hot white rice (see Tip, left).

AMERICA'S EXCHANGES	
2	Medium-fat Meat

CANADA'S CHOICES	
2	Meat and Alternatives
1	Fat

MAKES 10 SERVINGS
(1 piece of chicken with
prunes and quinoa per
serving)

Tips

Some quinoa has a resinous coating called saponin, which needs to be rinsed off. To ensure your quinoa is saponin-free, before cooking fill a bowl with warm water and swish the kernels around, then transfer to a sieve and rinse thoroughly under cold running water.

If you are marinating the chicken overnight, refrigerate the prune mixture.

Moroccan-Style Chicken with Prunes and Quinoa

A variation on a traditional Moroccan tagine, this delicious dish makes the most of the bittersweet combination of prunes, honey and lemon. The addition of garlic, oregano and a smattering of black pepper completes the flavor profile. Traditionally, this dish is served with couscous, but I've used quinoa, which is every bit as tasty and more nutritious.

- **Works in slow cookers from 3½ to 6 quarts**

1½ cups	chopped pitted prunes	375 mL
1½ cups	water	375 mL
1 tbsp	liquid honey	15 mL
1 tsp	grated lemon zest	5 mL
4	cloves garlic, minced	4
1 tbsp	dried oregano leaves, crumbled	15 mL
1 tbsp	grated lemon zest	15 mL
½ tsp	salt	2 mL
½ tsp	cracked black peppercorns	2 mL
2½ lbs	skinless bone-in chicken thighs (about 10 thighs)	1.25 kg
2 cups	lower-salt chicken broth	500 mL
¼ cup	freshly squeezed lemon juice	50 mL
3 cups	water	750 mL
1½ cups	quinoa, rinsed (see Tips, left)	375 mL

1. In a bowl, combine prunes, the 1½ cups (375 mL) water, honey and lemon zest. Cover and set aside (see Tips, left).

2. In slow cooker stoneware, combine garlic, oregano, lemon zest, salt and peppercorns. Add chicken and toss until evenly coated with mixture. Cover and refrigerate for at least 1 hour or overnight.

3. Add broth and lemon juice to stoneware and stir well. Cover and cook on Low for 5 hours or on High for 2½ hours, until juices run clear when chicken is pierced with a fork. Add prunes with liquid. Cover and cook on High for 30 minutes to meld flavors.

NUTRIENTS PER SERVING	
Calories	265
Fat	5.6 g
Saturates	1.3 g
Polyunsaturates	1.5 g
Monounsaturates	2.0 g
Cholesterol	53 mg
Sodium	276 mg
Carbohydrate	36.7 g
Fiber	4.0 g
Protein	18.5 g

AMERICA'S EXCHANGES	
1	Starch
1½	Fruit
2	Lean Meat

CANADA'S CHOICES	
2	Carbohydrate
2	Meat and Alternatives

Make Ahead

This dish can be partially prepared before it is cooked. Complete Steps 1 and 2. Cover and refrigerate overnight or for up to 2 days. When you're ready to cook, continue with Steps 3 through 5.

4. Meanwhile, in a pot over high heat, bring the 3 cups (750 mL) water to a boil. Reduce heat to medium. Add quinoa in a steady stream, stirring to prevent lumps from forming, and return to a boil. Cover, reduce heat to low and simmer until tender and liquid is absorbed, about 15 minutes. Set aside.

5. To serve, spoon quinoa onto a plate and top with chicken mixture.

Mindful Morsels

Nutritionally, prunes have much to offer. Prunes are a source of potassium, which helps to keep blood pressure under control when consumed as part of a nutritious, balanced diet. Prunes also contain antioxidant phenols and beta carotene. Prunes are best known as an excellent source of fiber. Just $\frac{1}{4}$ cup (50 mL) of prunes contains 3 g of dietary fiber, which is associated with a wide range of healthful benefits, in addition to keeping you regular. Prunes also have a low glycemic index, which is good news for people with diabetes.

Tips

Cumin, a spice with a unique peppery yet earthy flavor, is used liberally in many cuisines.

If you don't have a 14-oz (398 mL) can of diced tomatoes, use 2 cups (500 mL) canned tomatoes with juice, coarsely chopped.

If using fresh spinach, be sure to remove the stems, and if it has not been pre-washed, rinse it thoroughly in a basin of lukewarm water. You will need to push it well down in the blender or food processor before puréeing in batches. If using frozen spinach, thaw it first and squeeze the water out.

One chile produces a medium-hot result. Add a second chile only if you're a true heat seeker.

Indian-Style Chicken with Puréed Spinach

This mouth-watering dish is an adaptation of one of my favorite recipes from Suneeta Vaswani's terrific book Easy Indian Cooking. *I usually serve it as the centerpiece of a meal, accompanied by rice and/or whole wheat chapati.*

- **Large (minimum 5 quart) oval slow cooker**

4 lbs	skinless bone-in chicken thighs (about 16 thighs)	2 kg
¼ cup	freshly squeezed lemon juice	50 mL
1 tbsp	cumin seeds (see Tips, left)	15 mL
2 tsp	coriander seeds	10 mL
2 tbsp	olive oil	25 mL
2	onions, thinly sliced on the vertical	2
1 tbsp	minced peeled gingerroot	15 mL
1 tbsp	minced garlic	15 mL
1 tsp	turmeric	5 mL
1 tsp	cracked black peppercorns	5 mL
½ tsp	salt	2 mL
1	can (14 oz/398 mL) diced tomatoes, including juice (see Tips, left)	1
2	packages (each 10 oz/300 g) fresh or frozen spinach (see Tips, left)	2
1 to 2	long red or green chile peppers, chopped (see Tips, left)	1 to 2
1 cup	lower-salt chicken broth	250 mL
	Juice of 1 lime or lemon	

1. Rinse chicken under cold running water and pat dry. In a bowl, combine chicken and lemon juice. Toss well and set aside for 20 to 30 minutes.

2. In a dry skillet over medium heat, toast cumin and coriander seeds, stirring, until fragrant and cumin seeds just begin to brown, about 3 minutes. Immediately transfer to a mortar or a spice grinder and grind. Set aside.

3. In same skillet, heat oil over medium-high heat for 30 seconds. Add onions and cook, stirring, until they begin to color, about 5 minutes. Reduce heat to medium and cook, stirring, until golden, about 12 minutes. Add reserved cumin and coriander, gingerroot, garlic, turmeric, peppercorns and salt and cook, stirring, for 1 minute. Stir in tomatoes with juice and bring to a boil. Remove from heat.

NUTRIENTS PER SERVING	
Calories	124
Fat	5.5 g
Saturates	1.3 g
Polyunsaturates	1.1 g
Monounsaturates	2.6 g
Cholesterol	48 mg
Sodium	214 mg
Carbohydrate	4.6 g
Fiber	1.6 g
Protein	14.2

AMERICA'S EXCHANGES	
1	Vegetable
2	Lean Meat

CANADA'S CHOICES	
2	Meat and Alternatives
1	Extra

Make Ahead

This dish can be partially prepared before it is cooked. Complete Step 1. Cover and refrigerate chicken. Complete Steps 2 and 3. Cover and refrigerate separately from chicken. The next day, continue with Steps 4 and 5.

4. Arrange marinated chicken evenly over the bottom of the slow cooker stoneware. Pour tomato mixture over top. Cover and cook on Low for 6 hours or on High for 3 hours, until juices run clear when chicken is pierced with a fork.

5. In a blender or food processor, combine spinach, chile(s) and broth. Pulse until spinach is puréed. Add to chicken and stir well. Cover and cook on High for 20 minutes, until mixture is bubbly. Just before serving, stir in lime juice.

Mindful Morsels

The spinach in this recipe provides over 100% of the daily value of vitamin K, which is found in many leafy greens and some vegetable oils, such as olive oil. Vitamin K is an important blood clotting agent and also plays a role in bone health.

MAKES 12 SERVINGS
(1 piece of chicken with
sauce per serving)

Tip

Buy seeds and nuts at a health
or bulk food store with high
turnover, as they are likely to be
much fresher than those in
packages.

Mexican-Style Chicken with Cilantro and Lemon

*With a sauce of pumpkin seeds, cumin seeds, oregano and cilantro,
this dish reminds me of warm evening dinners in the courtyard of a
charming Mexican hacienda. Mexicans have been thickening
sauces with pumpkin seeds since long before the Spanish arrived
and, today, every cook has his or her own recipe for mole, one of the
world's great culinary concoctions. Serve this with rice and fresh
corn on the cob.*

• **Works in slow cookers from 3½ to 6 quarts**

¼ cup	raw pumpkin seeds	50 mL
2 tsp	cumin seeds	10 mL
1 tbsp	olive oil	15 mL
2	onions, sliced	2
4	cloves garlic, minced	4
2 tbsp	tomato paste	25 mL
1 tsp	salt	5 mL
1 tsp	cracked black peppercorns	5 mL
1 tsp	dried oregano leaves	5 mL
¼ tsp	ground cinnamon	1 mL
1 cup	coarsely chopped cilantro, stems and leaves	250 mL
1 tbsp	grated lemon zest	15 mL
2 tbsp	freshly squeezed lemon juice	25 mL
½ cup	lower-salt chicken broth	125 mL
3 lbs	skinless bone-in chicken thighs (about 12 thighs)	1.5 kg
1 to 2	jalapeño peppers, chopped	1 to 2
	Finely chopped cilantro and green onion	
	Grated lemon zest	

1. In a skillet, over medium-high heat, toast pumpkin and cumin seeds, stirring constantly, until pumpkin seeds are popping and cumin is fragrant, about 3 minutes. Transfer to a small bowl and set aside.

2. In the same skillet, heat oil over medium heat for 30 seconds. Add onions to pan and cook, stirring, until softened, about 3 minutes. Add garlic, tomato paste, salt, peppercorns, oregano and cinnamon and cook, stirring, for 1 minute. Transfer contents of pan to a blender or food processor. Add cilantro, lemon zest and juice, broth and reserved pumpkin and cumin seeds and process until smooth.

NUTRIENTS PER SERVING	
Calories	126
Fat	5.4 g
Saturates	1.3 g
Polyunsaturates	1.1 g
Monounsaturates	2.4 g
Cholesterol	53 mg
Sodium	271 mg
Carbohydrate	4.3 g
Fiber	0.9 g
Protein	14.8 g

AMERICA'S EXCHANGES	
2	Lean Meat

CANADA'S CHOICES	
2	Meat and Alternatives

Make Ahead

This dish can be partially prepared before it is cooked. Complete Steps 1 and 2. Cover and refrigerate puréed sauce overnight. The next morning, continue with the recipe.

3. Arrange chicken over bottom of slow cooker stoneware and cover with vegetable mixture. Cover and cook on Low for 6 hours or on High for 3 hours, until juices run clear when chicken is pierced with a fork. Stir in jalapeño peppers. When you're ready to serve, garnish with cilantro, green onion and lemon zest.

Mindful Morsels

Culinary herbs do more than add color and flavor to a dish: they also have health benefits. For instance, USDA researchers have found that many culinary herbs, such as sage, dill, thyme and rosemary, are loaded with antioxidants, a group of nutrients that protect your body against the harmful effects of free radicals, much like rust-proofing protects your car from rust. Recent research suggests that the best way to consume antioxidants is in food, where they work together as part of the whole food. Some studies have shown that taking antioxidants as supplements does not produce similar benefits.

MAKES 8 SERVINGS
(about 2¹/₂ oz/75 g turkey
with sauce per serving)

Make Ahead

This dish can be partially
prepared before it is cooked.
Complete Steps 1 and 3. Cover
and refrigerate for up to 2 days.
When you're ready to cook,
heat 1 tbsp (15 mL) oil in pan
and brown turkey breast
(Step 2), or if you're pressed
for time, remove skin from
turkey breast, omit browning
and place directly in slow cooker
stoneware. If you are not
browning the turkey, omit
the optional brandy flambé.
Continue with the recipe.

Best-Ever Turkey Breast

*If you want to celebrate a holiday with turkey but don't feel like
cooking an entire bird, try this tasty alternative. Accompany with
roast or mashed potatoes, Brussels sprouts and cranberry ketchup for
a great festive meal.*

- **Works best in a large (minimum 5 quart) slow cooker**

2	slices bacon	2
2 tbsp	olive oil	25 mL
1	skin-on turkey breast (about 2 lbs/1 kg)	1
2 tbsp	brandy or cognac, optional	25 mL
2	onions, finely chopped	2
4	carrots, peeled and diced	4
4	stalks celery, diced	4
2	cloves garlic, minced	2
1 tsp	ground sage	5 mL
6	whole cloves or allspice	6
1 tsp	salt	5 mL
¹/₂ tsp	cracked black peppercorns	2 mL
¹/₄ cup	all-purpose flour	50 mL
³/₄ cup	dry white wine or lower-salt chicken broth	175 mL

1. In a skillet, cook bacon over medium-high heat until crisp. Remove from pan and drain on paper towel. Crumble and set aside. Drain fat from pan. Add oil.

2. Add turkey breast to pan and brown on all sides. Turn turkey skin side up and sprinkle with brandy, if using. Ignite, stand back and wait for flames to subside. Transfer to slow cooker stoneware.

3. Reduce heat to medium. Add onions, carrots and celery to pan and cook, stirring, until vegetables are softened, about 7 minutes. Add garlic, sage, cloves, salt and peppercorns and cook, stirring, for 1 minute. Sprinkle flour over mixture and cook, stirring, for 1 minute. Stir in reserved bacon and wine and cook, stirring, until mixture is thickened.

4. Spoon sauce over turkey breast. Cover and cook on Low for 6 hours or on High for 3 hours, until turkey is tender and no longer pink inside or an instant-read meat thermometer reads 170°F (77°C). Transfer turkey to a warm platter, spoon sauce over and serve piping hot.

NUTRIENTS PER SERVING	
Calories	201
Fat	6.8 g
Saturates	2.0 g
Polyunsaturates	1.6 g
Monounsaturates	2.3 g
Cholesterol	59 mg
Sodium	404 mg
Carbohydrate	9.6 g
Fiber	1.6 g
Protein	24.2 g

AMERICA'S EXCHANGES	
2	Vegetable
3	Lean Meat

CANADA'S CHOICES	
¹/₂	Carbohydrate
3	Meat and Alternatives

Tips

If you don't have hot paprika, use regular paprika instead with a pinch of cayenne.

If you don't have a mortar or a spice grinder, place the toasted fennel seeds on a cutting board and use the bottom of a wine bottle or measuring cup to grind them.

Make Ahead

This dish can be partially prepared before it is cooked. Complete Steps 1 and 2. Cover and refrigerate overnight or for up to 2 days. When you're ready to cook, continue with Step 3.

Turkey, Mushroom and Chickpea Sauce

Kids always want seconds of this lip-smacking sauce, which is delicious over chunky pasta, brown rice or polenta. For a change, try it over hot quinoa, whose New World origins resonate with turkey.

- **Works in slow cookers from 3½ to 6 quarts**

½ tsp	fennel seeds	2 mL
1 tbsp	olive oil	15 mL
1 lb	ground turkey	500 g
2	onions, minced	2
4	stalks celery, diced	4
2	cloves garlic, minced	2
1 tsp	dried oregano leaves, crumbled	5 mL
½ tsp	cracked black peppercorns	2 mL
8 oz	cremini mushrooms, trimmed and quartered	250 g
1	can (28 oz/796 mL) diced tomatoes, including juice	1
1 cup	lower-salt vegetable or chicken broth	250 mL
1	can (14 oz/398 mL) chickpeas, drained and rinsed	1
2 tsp	hot paprika (see Tips, left), dissolved in 1 tbsp (15 mL) lemon juice	10 mL
1	red bell pepper, diced	1

1. In a dry skillet over medium heat, toast fennel seeds, stirring, until fragrant, about 3 minutes. Immediately transfer to a mortar or a spice grinder and grind (see Tips, left). Set aside.

2. In same skillet, heat oil over medium heat for 30 seconds. Add turkey, onions and celery and cook, stirring, until celery is softened and no hint of pink remains in the turkey, about 6 minutes. Add fennel seeds, garlic, oregano and peppercorns and cook, stirring, for 1 minute. Add mushrooms and toss to coat. Add tomatoes, with juice, and broth and bring to a boil. Transfer to slow cooker stoneware. Add chickpeas and stir well.

3. Cover and cook on Low for 6 hours or on High for 3 hours, until mixture is hot and bubbly. Add paprika solution and stir well. Add bell pepper and stir well. Cover and cook on High for 20 minutes, until pepper is tender.

NUTRIENTS PER SERVING	
Calories	260
Fat	9.6 g
Saturates	2.2 g
Polyunsaturates	2.2 g
Monounsaturates	4.2 g
Cholesterol	60 mg
Sodium	397 mg
Carbohydrate	26.5 g
Fiber	5.7 g
Protein	19.0 g

AMERICA'S EXCHANGES	
1	Starch
2	Vegetable
2	Lean Meat
½	Fat

CANADA'S CHOICES	
1½	Carbohydrate
2	Meat and Alternatives

Tips

Canned tomatoes vary in sizes. If your supermarket carries the 19-oz (540 mL) can of diced tomatoes, by all means substitute it in this recipe.

For convenience, use bottled roasted red peppers or, if you prefer, roast your own.

Some quinoa has a resinous coating called saponin, which needs to be rinsed off. To ensure your quinoa is saponin-free, before cooking fill a bowl with warm water and swish the kernels around, then transfer to a sieve and rinse thoroughly under cold running water.

Variation

Peppery Turkey Stew: Omit the quinoa. Serve the stew over hot rice or mashed potatoes.

Peppery Turkey Casserole

With five different kinds of peppers, this dish is a testament to the depth and variety of this useful ingredient. I've added quinoa because it's so nutritious and isn't commonly included in the North American diet. Here, I've stirred it in after the dish has finished cooking to make a casserole, but if you prefer, serve it on the side.

- **Works in slow cookers from 3½ to 6 quarts**

1 tbsp	olive oil	15 mL
2	onions, finely chopped	2
4	cloves garlic, minced	4
2 tsp	dried oregano leaves, crumbled	10 mL
½ tsp	cracked black peppercorns	2 mL
1 cup	dry white wine	250 mL
1	can (14 oz/398 mL) diced tomatoes, including juice (see Tips, left)	1
2 cups	lower-salt chicken broth	500 mL
1½ lbs	bone-in turkey breast, skin removed, cut into ½-inch (1 cm) cubes (about 2½ cups/625 mL)	750 g
2 tsp	sweet paprika, dissolved in 2 tbsp (25 mL) water	10 mL
1	jalapeño pepper, finely chopped	1
2	green bell peppers, diced	2
1	roasted red bell pepper, diced (see Tips, left)	1
3 cups	water	750 mL
1½ cups	quinoa, rinsed (see Tips, left)	375 mL

1. In a skillet, heat oil over medium heat for 30 seconds. Add onions and cook, stirring, until softened, about 3 minutes. Add garlic, oregano and peppercorns and cook, stirring, for 1 minute. Add white wine and tomatoes with juice and bring to a boil. Transfer to slow cooker stoneware. Add broth and stir well.

2. Add turkey and stir well. Cover and cook on Low for 6 hours or on High for 3 hours, until turkey is tender.

3. Add paprika solution, jalapeño pepper, bell peppers and roasted red pepper to slow cooker stoneware and stir well. Cover and cook on High for 30 minutes, until peppers are tender.

NUTRIENTS PER SERVING	
Calories	256
Fat	5.2 g
Saturates	0.9 g
Polyunsaturates	1.3 g
Monounsaturates	2.3 g
Cholesterol	37 mg
Sodium	385 mg
Carbohydrate	30.5 g
Fiber	3.5 g
Protein	22.2 g

AMERICA'S EXCHANGES	
1½	Starch
1	Vegetable
2	Lean Meat

CANADA'S CHOICES	
2	Carbohydrate
2	Meat and Alternatives

This dish can be partially prepared before it is cooked. Complete Step 1. Cover and refrigerate overnight or for up to 2 days. When you're ready to cook, continue with Steps 2 through 5.

4. Meanwhile, in a pot, bring water to a boil. Add quinoa in a steady stream, stirring to prevent lumps from forming, and return to a boil. Cover, reduce heat to low and simmer until tender and liquid is absorbed, about 15 minutes. Set aside.

5. When peppers are tender, add cooked quinoa to slow cooker stoneware and stir well. Serve immediately.

Mindful Morsels

A serving of this dish provides about 30% of the daily value of vitamin B_6. The bell peppers and the turkey are a source of this vitamin, which is best known for keeping skin healthy. But B_6 plays a role in keeping your mind sharp and it boosts serotonin, which helps to keep depression at bay. It also helps your body make new cells to produce infection-fighting antibodies and may lower the risk of colon cancer, one of the most common cancers in North America.

Turkey Mole

Make Ahead

This dish can be partially prepared before it is cooked. Complete Steps 2 and 4, heating 1 tbsp (15 mL) oil in pan before softening onions. Cover and refrigerate puréed sauces separately for up to 2 days, being aware that the chile mixture will lose some of its vibrancy if held for this long. (For best results, complete Step 4 while the turkey is cooking or no sooner than the night before you plan to cook.) When you're ready to cook, brown turkey (Step 1), or remove skin from turkey, omit browning and place directly in stoneware. Continue with the recipe.

In many parts of Mexico, no special occasion is complete without turkey cooked in mole poblano. Since the authentic version is quite a production, I've simplified this slow cooker version, which is delicious nonetheless. Serve with hot tortillas, fluffy rice and creamed corn.

• **Works best in a large (minimum 5 quart) slow cooker**

1 tbsp	olive oil	15 mL
1	skin-on turkey breast (about 2 lbs/1 kg)	1
2	onions, sliced	2
4	cloves garlic, sliced	4
4	whole cloves	4
1	piece (2 inches/5 cm) cinnamon stick	1
1 tsp	salt	5 mL
1 tsp	cracked black peppercorns	5 mL
1	can (28 oz/796 mL) tomatillos, drained	1
1/2 oz	unsweetened chocolate, broken in pieces	15 g
1 cup	lower-salt chicken broth, divided	250 mL
2	dried ancho, New Mexico or guajillo chiles	2
2 cups	boiling water	500 mL
1/2 cup	coarsely chopped cilantro stems and leaves	125 mL
1 tbsp	chili powder	15 mL
1 to 2	jalapeño peppers, chopped	1 to 2
3 tbsp	diced mild green chiles, optional	45 mL

1. In a skillet, heat oil over medium-high heat for 30 seconds. Add turkey and brown on all sides. Transfer to slow cooker stoneware.

2. Reduce heat to medium. Add onions to pan and cook, stirring, until softened, about 3 minutes. Add garlic, cloves, cinnamon stick, salt and peppercorns and cook, stirring, for 1 minute. Transfer mixture to blender. Add tomatillos, chocolate and 1/2 cup (125 mL) of the broth and process until smooth.

3. Pour sauce over turkey, cover and cook on Low for 8 hours or on High for 4 hours, until juices run clear when turkey is pierced with a fork or meat thermometer reads 170°F (77°C).

NUTRIENTS PER SERVING	
Calories	224
Fat	9.8 g
Saturates	2.6 g
Polyunsaturates	2.2 g
Monounsaturates	3.6 g
Cholesterol	58 mg
Sodium	418 mg
Carbohydrate	10.4 g
Fiber	2.1 g
Protein	24.7 g

AMERICA'S EXCHANGES	
2	Vegetable
3	Lean Meat

CANADA'S CHOICES	
1/2	Carbohydrate
3	Meat and Alternatives

4. Half an hour before recipe has finished cooking, in a heatproof bowl, soak dried chiles in boiling water for 30 minutes, weighing down with a cup to ensure they remain submerged. Drain, discarding soaking liquid and stems, and chop coarsely. Transfer to a blender. Add cilantro, remaining $\frac{1}{2}$ cup (125 mL) of the broth, chili powder and jalapeño pepper and purée. Add to stoneware along with mild green chiles, if using, and stir gently to combine. Cover and cook on High for 30 minutes, until flavors meld.

Mindful Morsels

Turkey is an excellent source of complete protein because, once the skin is removed, it is a very lean meat. In addition to being rich in protein, turkey is a good source of important B vitamins — niacin, B_6 and B_{12} — as well as zinc, which helps to keep your immune system strong. Turkey is also a good source of the trace mineral selenium, which acts as an antioxidant.

MAKES 6 SERVINGS
(about 2½ oz/75 g turkey
with sauce per serving)

Tips

I've left the skin on the turkey breast and browned it before cooking to more closely approximate the result of a traditional roast turkey.

To clean leeks: Fill a sink full of lukewarm water. Split the leeks in half lengthwise and submerge them in the water, swishing them around to remove all traces of dirt. Transfer to a colander and rinse thoroughly under cold water.

Make Ahead

This dish can be partially prepared before it is cooked. Heat oil and complete Step 2. Cover and refrigerate overnight or for up to 2 days. When you're ready to cook, complete Steps 1 and 3.

Turkey in Cranberry Leek Sauce

Here's a simple, yet delicious treatment for a whole turkey breast. Serve this with mashed potatoes and steamed green beans for a traditional comfort food meal, or substitute a whole grain, such as brown rice or quinoa.

- **Large (minimum 5 quart) slow cooker**
- **Instant-read thermometer**

1 tbsp	olive oil	15 mL
1	skin-on bone-in turkey breast (about 1½ lbs/750 g) (see Tip, left)	1
2	medium leeks, white part only with just a bit of green, cleaned and thinly sliced (see Tip, left)	2
2	cloves garlic, minced	2
2 tsp	dried thyme leaves	10 mL
½ tsp	cracked black peppercorns	2 mL
1 tbsp	all-purpose flour	15 mL
1 cup	lower-salt chicken broth	250 mL
½ cup	dried cranberries	125 mL
2 tbsp	finely chopped parsley	25 mL

1. In a skillet, heat oil over medium-high heat for 30 seconds. Add turkey breast, skin side down, and cook until nicely browned, about 4 minutes. Transfer, skin side up, to slow cooker stoneware.

2. Reduce heat to medium. Add leeks and cook, stirring, until softened, about 5 minutes. Add garlic, thyme and peppercorns and cook, stirring, for 1 minute. Add flour and cook, stirring, for 1 minute. Add broth and cook, stirring, until mixture begins to thicken, about 2 minutes. Stir in cranberries.

3. Transfer sauce to slow cooker stoneware, covering turkey with sauce. Cover and cook on Low for 5½ to 6 hours or on High for 2½ to 3 hours, until an instant-read thermometer inserted into center of breast registers 175°F (80°C). To serve, transfer to a platter and garnish with parsley.

NUTRIENTS PER SERVING	
Calories	218
Fat	8.5 g
Saturates	1.9 g
Polyunsaturates	1.5 g
Monounsaturates	4.2 g
Cholesterol	54 mg
Sodium	166 mg
Carbohydrate	13.2 g
Fiber	1.8 g
Protein	21.7 g

AMERICA'S EXCHANGES	
½	Fruit
1	Vegetable
3	Lean Meat

CANADA'S CHOICES	
1	Carbohydrate
3	Meat and Alternatives

Meat

Tip

While round steak is traditionally used for this dish, an equally successful version can be made with "simmering steak." This is cut from the blade or cross rib and is available at many supermarkets.

Make Ahead

This dish can be partially prepared before it is cooked. Complete Step 2, heating 1 tbsp (15 mL) oil in pan before softening onions, carrots and celery. Cover and refrigerate mixture for up to 2 days. When you're ready to cook, brown steak (Step 1), or omit this step and place steak directly in stoneware. Continue cooking as directed. Alternatively, cook steak overnight, cover and refrigerate. When ready to serve, bring to a boil in a large skillet and simmer for 10 minutes, until meat is heated through and sauce is hot and bubbly.

Saucy Swiss Steak

Here's a dish that many people will remember from the 1950s. Back then it required a fair bit of muscle to pound the steak with a mallet. Today, you can avoid all that dreary work by using the slow cooker. Serve with garlic mashed potatoes and a plain green vegetable.

- **Large (minimum 5 quart) slow cooker**

1 tbsp	olive oil	15 mL
2 lbs	round steak or "simmering" steak (see Tip, left), trimmed of fat	1 kg
2	onions, finely chopped	2
1	carrot, peeled and thinly sliced	1
1	stalk celery, thinly sliced	1
½ tsp	salt	2 mL
¼ tsp	cracked black peppercorns	1 mL
2 tbsp	all-purpose flour	25 mL
1	can (28 oz/796 mL) diced tomatoes, drained, ½ cup (125 mL) juice reserved	1
1 tbsp	Worcestershire sauce	15 mL
1	bay leaf	1

1. In a skillet, heat oil over medium-high heat for 30 seconds. Add steak, in pieces, if necessary, and brown on both sides. Transfer to slow cooker stoneware.

2. Reduce heat to medium-low. Add onions, carrot, celery, salt and peppercorns to pan. Cover and cook until carrots are softened, about 7 minutes. Sprinkle flour over vegetables and cook, stirring, for 1 minute. Add tomatoes, reserved juice and Worcestershire sauce. Bring to a boil, stirring until slightly thickened. Add bay leaf.

3. Pour tomato mixture over steak. Cover and cook on Low for 8 hours or on for High 4 hours, until meat is tender. Discard bay leaf.

NUTRIENTS PER SERVING	
Calories	142
Fat	3.9 g
Saturates	1.0 g
Polyunsaturates	0.3 g
Monounsaturates	1.9 g
Cholesterol	39 mg
Sodium	280 mg
Carbohydrate	6.8 g
Fiber	1.1 g
Protein	19.5 g

AMERICA'S EXCHANGES	
1	Vegetable
2½	Very Lean Meat

CANADA'S CHOICES	
½	Carbohydrate
2½	Meat and Alternatives

Tip

While round steak is traditionally used for this dish, an equally successful version can be made with "simmering steak." This is cut from the blade or cross rib and is available at many supermarkets.

Make Ahead

This dish can be partially prepared before it is cooked. Complete Step 2, heating 1 tbsp (15 mL) oil in pan before softening onions. Cover and refrigerate mixture for up to 2 days. When you're ready to cook, brown steak (Step 1), or omit this step and place meat directly in stoneware. Continue with the recipe.

NUTRIENTS PER SERVING	
Calories	193
Fat	7.4 g
Saturates	2.9 g
Polyunsaturates	0.4 g
Monounsaturates	3.2 g
Cholesterol	59 mg
Sodium	381 mg
Carbohydrate	6.4 g
Fiber	0.8 g
Protein	24.1 g

Ranch House Chicken Fried Steak

There's no chicken in it, so where did this classic cowboy dish get its name? Frankly, who cares? Making it in the slow cooker eliminates the traditional tasks of pounding the meat and watching the frying pan. It also produces melt-in-your-mouth results. The rich, spicy pan gravy served over mashed potatoes is a marriage made in heaven. To turn up the heat, increase the quantity of jalapeño pepper.

- **Large (minimum 5 quart) slow cooker**

1 tbsp	olive oil	15 mL
2 lbs	round steak or "simmering" steak (see Tip, left), trimmed of fat	1 kg
2	onions, thinly sliced	2
3	cloves garlic, minced	3
1 tsp	salt	5 mL
1 tsp	cracked black peppercorns	5 mL
1/4 cup	all-purpose flour	50 mL
3/4 cup	lower-salt chicken broth	175 mL
1 tsp	paprika	5 mL
1/4 tsp	cayenne pepper	1 mL
1/4 cup	whipping (35%) cream	50 mL
1 to 2	jalapeño peppers, finely chopped	1 to 2
	Hot fluffy mashed potatoes	

1. In a skillet, heat oil over medium-high heat for 30 seconds. Add steak, in pieces, if necessary, and brown on both sides. Transfer to slow cooker stoneware.

2. Reduce heat to medium. Add onions to skillet and cook, stirring, until softened, about 3 minutes. Add garlic, salt and peppercorns and cook, stirring, for 1 minute. Sprinkle flour over mixture and cook, stirring, for 1 minute. Add broth and cook, stirring, until thickened. (Sauce will be very thick.)

3. Spoon sauce over meat in slow cooker, cover and cook on Low for 8 hours or on High for 4 hours, until meat is tender.

4. In a small bowl, combine paprika and cayenne. Gradually add cream, mixing until blended. Add to stoneware along with jalapeño pepper. Cover and cook on High for 15 minutes, until flavors meld. Serve with hot fluffy mashed potatoes.

AMERICA'S EXCHANGES	
1/2	Other Carbohydrate
3	Lean Meat

CANADA'S CHOICES	
1/2	Carbohydrate
3	Meat and Alternatives

Classic Beef Stew

Here's an old-fashioned stew that is simply delicious.

Make Ahead

This stew can be partially prepared before it is cooked. Complete Step 2, heating 1 tbsp (15 mL) oil in skillet before softening the vegetables. Cover and refrigerate for up to 2 days. When you're ready to cook, brown the meat (Step 1), or if you're pressed for time, omit this step and place the meat directly in the stoneware. Continue with the recipe.

- **Large (minimum 5 quart) slow cooker**

1 tbsp	olive oil	15 mL
2 lbs	trimmed stewing beef, cut into 1-inch (2.5 cm) cubes	1 kg
2	large onions, finely chopped	2
4	stalks celery, diced	4
2	large carrots, peeled and diced	2
2	cloves garlic, minced	2
1 tsp	dried thyme leaves	5 mL
1 tsp	salt	5 mL
½ tsp	cracked black peppercorns	2 mL
¼ cup	all-purpose flour	50 mL
1 cup	lower-salt beef broth	250 mL
½ cup	dry red wine or additional lower-salt beef broth	125 mL
2	bay leaves	2
	Finely chopped fresh parsley	

1. In a skillet, heat half the oil over medium-high heat for 30 seconds. Add beef, in batches, and cook, stirring, adding remaining oil as necessary, until lightly browned, about 4 minutes per batch. Using a slotted spoon, transfer to slow cooker stoneware.

2. Reduce heat to medium. Add onions, celery and carrots and cook, stirring, until vegetables are softened, about 7 minutes. Add garlic, thyme, salt and peppercorns and cook, stirring, for 1 minute. Add flour and cook, stirring, for 1 minute. Add broth and wine and cook, stirring, until thickened. Add bay leaves.

3. Transfer mixture to slow cooker stoneware and stir thoroughly to combine ingredients. Cover and cook on Low for 8 to 10 hours or on High for 4 to 5 hours, until beef is very tender. Discard bay leaves. Just before serving, garnish liberally with parsley.

NUTRIENTS PER SERVING	
Calories	212
Fat	8.8 g
Saturates	2.8 g
Polyunsaturates	0.6 g
Monounsaturates	3.9 g
Cholesterol	47 mg
Sodium	516 mg
Carbohydrate	9.3 g
Fiber	1.4 g
Protein	22.9 g

AMERICA'S EXCHANGES	
2	Vegetable
3	Lean Meat

CANADA'S CHOICES	
½	Carbohydrate
3	Meat and Alternatives

Tips

To peel pearl onions, cut a small "x" in the bottom and drop in a pot of boiling water for 1 minute. Drain and rinse under cold running water. The skins will come off easily with a paring knife.

The little bit of sugar in this recipe nicely balances the acidity of the vinegar. If you prefer not to use sugar, you may substitute your favorite low-calorie sweetener.

Make Ahead

This dish can be partially prepared before it is cooked. Complete Step 2, heating 1 tbsp (15 mL) oil in pan before softening onions. Cover and refrigerate mixture for up to 2 days. When you're ready to cook, brown beef (Step 1), or if you're pressed for time, omit this step and add meat directly to stoneware. Continue cooking as directed in Steps 3 and 4.

Greek Beef Stew with Onions and Feta

This robust stew, known as stifado in Greece, is different and delicious. The feta and vinegar add tartness, which is nicely balanced by a tiny bit of sugar, along with cinnamon and allspice. Use only good-quality tomato sauce and serve as Greek people do, with long strands of hot buttered macaroni, often known as bucatini (not the usual broken or stubby variety), or fluffy mashed potatoes.

- **Large (minimum 5 quart) slow cooker**

1 tbsp	olive oil	15 mL
2 lbs	trimmed stewing beef, cut into 1-inch (2.5 cm) cubes	1 kg
3	large onions, finely chopped, or 2 lbs (1 kg) pearl onions (see Tips, left)	3
4	cloves garlic, minced	4
1/2 tsp	ground cinnamon	2 mL
1/2 tsp	ground allspice	2 mL
1 1/2 cups	tomato sauce	375 mL
3 tbsp	red wine vinegar	45 mL
1 tsp	granulated sugar	5 mL
1	bay leaf	1
1/2 cup	crumbled light feta cheese	125 mL
	Macaroni, noodles or mashed potatoes	

1. In a skillet, heat half the oil over medium-high heat for 30 seconds. Add beef, in batches, and cook, stirring, adding remaining oil as necessary, until lightly browned, about 4 minutes per batch. Using a slotted spoon, transfer to slow cooker stoneware.

2. Reduce heat to medium. Add onions and cook, stirring, until softened, about 3 minutes. Add garlic, cinnamon and allspice and cook, stirring, for 1 minute. Add tomato sauce, vinegar, sugar and bay leaf and stir to combine.

3. Pour mixture over meat and cook on Low for 8 to 10 hours or on High for 4 to 5 hours, until beef is tender.

4. Add feta cheese and cook on High for 10 minutes. Discard bay leaf. Spoon over hot buttered macaroni, noodles or mashed potatoes.

NUTRIENTS PER SERVING	
Calories	228
Fat	10.2 g
Saturates	3.7 g
Polyunsaturates	0.6 g
Monounsaturates	3.8 g
Cholesterol	50 mg
Sodium	454 mg
Carbohydrate	9.7 g
Fiber	1.6 g
Protein	24.4 g

AMERICA'S EXCHANGES	
2	Vegetable
3	Lean Meat

CANADA'S CHOICES	
1/2	Carbohydrate
3	Meat and Alternatives

Tip

To cook bulgur to accompany this recipe, combine 2 cups (500 mL) medium or fine bulgur and 4 cups (1 L) boiling water. Cover and set aside until water is absorbed and bulgur is tender to the bite, about 20 minutes.

Greek-Style Beef with Eggplant

This ambrosial stew reminds me of moussaka without the topping, and it is far less work. Made with red wine and lycopene-rich tomato paste, it develops a deep and intriguing flavor. Serve this over hot bulgur (see Tip, left) and accompany with steamed broccoli and a tossed green salad for a delicious and nutrient-rich meal.

- **Works in slow cookers from 3½ to 6 quarts**
- **Large rimmed baking sheet**

2	medium eggplants (each about 1 lb/500 g) peeled, halved and each half cut into quarters	2
2 tbsp	kosher salt	25 mL
2 tbsp	olive oil, divided	25 mL
1 lb	lean ground beef	500 g
4	onions, thinly sliced on the vertical	4
4	cloves garlic, minced	4
2 tsp	dried oregano leaves, crumbled	10 mL
1 tsp	ground cinnamon	5 mL
½ tsp	salt	2 mL
½ tsp	cracked black peppercorns	2 mL
1	can (5½ oz/156 mL) tomato paste	1
1 cup	dry red wine	250 mL
1 cup	packed parsley leaves, finely chopped	250 mL
	Grated Parmesan cheese	

1. In a colander over a sink, combine eggplant and kosher salt. Toss to ensure eggplant is well coated and set aside for 30 minutes to 1 hour. Meanwhile, preheat oven to 400°F (200°C). Rinse eggplant well under cold running water and drain. Pat dry with paper towel. Brush all over with 1 tbsp (15 mL) of the oil. Place on baking sheet and bake until soft and fragrant, about 20 minutes. Transfer to slow cooker stoneware.

NUTRIENTS PER SERVING	
Calories	225
Fat	11.7 g
Saturates	3.7 g
Polyunsaturates	0.7 g
Monounsaturates	6.0 g
Cholesterol	34 mg
Sodium	204 mg
Carbohydrate	17.8 g
Fiber	4.8 g
Protein	13.9 g

AMERICA'S EXCHANGES	
1	Carbohydrate
1½	Lean Meat
1½	Fat

CANADA'S CHOICES	
1	Carbohydrate
1½	Meat and Alternatives
1	Fat

Make Ahead

This dish can be partially prepared before it is cooked. Complete Steps 1 and 2, placing eggplant and meat mixtures in separate containers. Cover and refrigerate overnight or for up to 2 days. When you're ready to cook, combine mixtures in stoneware and complete Step 3.

2. In a skillet, heat remaining 1 tbsp (15 mL) of the oil over medium heat for 30 seconds. Add ground beef and onions and cook, stirring and breaking up with a spoon, until beef is no longer pink, about 10 minutes. Add garlic, oregano, cinnamon, salt and peppercorns and cook, stirring, for 1 minute. Add tomato paste and red wine and stir well. Transfer to slow cooker stoneware. Stir well.

3. Cover and cook on Low for 8 hours or on High for 4 hours, until mixture is bubbly and eggplant is tender. Stir in parsley and serve. Pass the Parmesan at the table.

Mindful Morsels

I often use a fair bit of parsley in my recipes for two reasons: it's very tasty, and it's loaded with nutrients, such as vitamin K.

Tip

Large cans of tomatoes come in 28 oz (796 mL) and 35 oz (980 mL) sizes. For convenience, I've called for the 28 oz (796 mL) size in my recipes. If you're using the 35 oz (980 mL) size, drain off 1 cup (250 mL) liquid before adding to the recipe.

Country Stew with Fennel

Full of character, this robust beef stew, which is rooted in French country cooking, is the perfect antidote to a bone-chilling night. Don't worry if you're not a fan of anchovies — they add depth to the sauce and their taste is negligible in the finished dish. I like to serve this over quinoa or whole wheat couscous, liberally garnished with parsley, but mashed potatoes work well, too.

- **Large (minimum 5 quart) slow cooker**

½ tsp	fennel seeds	2 mL
1 tbsp	olive oil	15 mL
1½ lbs	trimmed stewing beef, cut into 1-inch (2.5 cm) cubes	750 g
2	onions, finely chopped	2
4	stalks celery, thinly sliced	4
1	bulb fennel, trimmed, cored and thinly sliced on the vertical	1
4	cloves garlic, minced	4
4	anchovy fillets, minced	4
1 tsp	dried thyme leaves	5 mL
¼ tsp	salt	1 mL
½ tsp	cracked black peppercorns	2 mL
1 tbsp	all-purpose flour	15 mL
1	can (28 oz/796 mL) diced tomatoes, including juice (see Tip, left)	1
2	bay leaves	2
½ cup	chopped pitted black olives	125 mL

1. In a dry skillet over medium heat, toast fennel seeds, stirring, until fragrant, about 3 minutes. Immediately transfer to a mortar or a spice grinder and grind. (Or place the seeds on a cutting board and crush, using the bottom of a bottle or cup.) Set aside.

2. In same skillet, heat half the oil over medium-high heat for 30 seconds. Add beef, in batches, and cook, stirring, adding remaining oil as necessary, until lightly browned, about 4 minutes per batch. Using a slotted spoon, transfer to slow cooker stoneware.

NUTRIENTS PER SERVING	
Calories	257
Fat	11.0 g
Saturates	3.1 g
Polyunsaturates	0.9 g
Monounsaturates	5.2 g
Cholesterol	49 mg
Sodium	624 mg
Carbohydrate	15.6 g
Fiber	3.7 g
Protein	24.9 g

AMERICA'S EXCHANGES	
3	Vegetable
3	Lean Meat

CANADA'S CHOICES	
1	Carbohydrate
3	Meat and Alternatives

Make Ahead

This dish can be partially prepared before it is cooked. Complete Step 1. Complete Step 3, heating 1 tbsp (15 mL) oil in pan before softening onions. Cover and refrigerate for up to 2 days. When you're ready to cook, either brown the beef as outlined in Step 2 or add it to the stoneware without browning. Stir well and continue with Step 4.

3. Reduce heat to medium. Add onions, celery and bulb fennel to pan and cook, stirring, until celery is softened, about 5 minutes. Add garlic, anchovies, thyme, salt, peppercorns and reserved fennel seeds and cook, stirring, for 1 minute. Add flour and cook, stirring, for 1 minute. Add tomatoes with juice and bring to a boil. Cook, stirring, just until mixture begins to thicken, about 2 minutes. Add bay leaves and stir well.

4. Transfer to slow cooker stoneware. Cover and cook on Low for 8 hours or on High for 4 hours, until beef is tender. Discard bay leaves. Stir in olives and serve.

Mindful Morsels

When cooking beef, trim as much of the visible fat as possible from the meat to reduce the calories and the amount of saturated fat you consume. About half the calories in untrimmed beef comes from the fat.

Tips

If you're using small mushrooms, quarter them. Large ones may be sliced.

To maximize your intake of nutrients when making this recipe, be sure to use whole (hulled) barley rather than pearl barley, from which the germ and most of the bran has been removed.

Count 1 tbsp (15 mL) of persillade as a Free Food/Extra.

Beef and Barley with Rosemary and Orange

This hearty stew, with its deep, rich flavors, makes a great family meal that is tasty enough to serve to company. Add a tossed green salad and a small crusty whole grain roll.

- **Large (minimum 5 quart) slow cooker**

2 tbsp	olive oil, divided	25 mL
2 lbs	trimmed stewing beef, cut into 1-inch (2.5 cm) cubes	1 kg
8 oz	mushrooms (see Tips, left)	250 g
3	onions, finely chopped	3
4	stalks celery, diced	4
4	carrots, peeled and diced	4
4	cloves garlic, minced	4
4	sprigs fresh rosemary or 2 tsp (10 mL) dried rosemary leaves, crumbled	4
1 tsp	cracked black peppercorns	5 mL
	Grated zest and juice of 1 orange	
1 cup	whole (hulled) or pot barley, rinsed (see Tips, left)	250 mL
3 cups	lower-salt beef broth	750 mL
1½ cups	dry red wine	375 mL

Persillade (optional)

1 cup	finely chopped parsley	250 mL
4	cloves garlic, minced	4
1 tsp	balsamic vinegar	5 mL

1. In a skillet, heat 1 tbsp (15 mL) of the oil over medium-high heat. Add beef, in batches, and cook, stirring, until browned, about 4 minutes per batch. Transfer to slow cooker stoneware.

2. Add remaining 1 tbsp (15 mL) of the oil to pan. Add mushrooms and toss until lightly seared, about 2 minutes. Transfer to slow cooker stoneware. Reduce heat to medium. Add onions, celery and carrots and cook, stirring, until carrots are softened, about 7 minutes. Add garlic, rosemary, peppercorns and orange zest and cook, stirring, for 1 minute. Add barley and toss to coat. Add orange juice, broth and wine and bring to a boil. Transfer to slow cooker stoneware. Stir well.

NUTRIENTS PER SERVING	
Calories	286
Fat	9.7 g
Saturates	2.8 g
Polyunsaturates	0.8 g
Monounsaturates	4.5 g
Cholesterol	44 mg
Sodium	387 mg
Carbohydrate	26.3 g
Fiber	3.7 g
Protein	23.7 g

AMERICA'S EXCHANGES	
1	Starch
2	Vegetable
3	Lean Meat

CANADA'S CHOICES	
1½	Carbohydrate
3	Meat and Alternatives

Make Ahead

This dish can be partially prepared before it is cooked. Complete Step 2. Cover and refrigerate overnight or for up to 2 days. When you're ready to cook, either brown the beef as outlined in Step 1 or add it to the stoneware without browning. Stir well and continue with Steps 3 and 4.

3. Cover and cook on Low for 8 hours or on High for 4 hours, until meat is tender.

4. **Persillade (optional):** In a bowl, combine parsley, garlic and vinegar. Set aside at room temperature for 30 minutes to allow flavors to develop. Ladle stew onto plates and garnish with persillade, if using.

If using fresh spinach, be sure to remove the stems, and if it has not been pre-washed, rinse it thoroughly in a basin of lukewarm water.

Beef and Chickpea Curry with Spinach

This combination of beef and chickpeas in an Indian-inspired sauce is particularly delicious. I like to serve this with long-grain brown rice, not only because I like its pleasant nutty flavor but also because it contains a significant amount of fiber. Complete this dinner with a platter of sliced tomatoes, in season, drizzled with olive oil and balsamic vinegar, or a green salad.

- **Works in slow cookers from 3½ to 6 quarts**

1 tbsp	olive oil	15 mL
1 lb	trimmed stewing beef, cut into ½-inch (1 cm) cubes	500 g
2	onions, finely chopped	2
4	cloves garlic, minced	4
1 tbsp	minced gingerroot	15 mL
½ tsp	cracked black peppercorns	2 mL
1	piece (1 inch/2.5 cm) cinnamon stick	1
1	bay leaf	1
1 cup	lower-salt beef broth	250 mL
1	can (14 to 19 oz/398 to 540 mL) chickpeas, drained and rinsed, or 1 cup (250 mL) dried chickpeas, soaked, cooked and drained (see Variation, page 231)	1
1 tsp	curry powder, dissolved in 2 tsp (10 mL) freshly squeezed lemon juice	5 mL
1 lb	fresh spinach, stems removed, or 1 package (10 oz/300 g) spinach leaves, thawed if frozen (see Tip, left)	500 g
	Low-fat plain yogurt, optional	

1. In a skillet, heat oil over medium-high heat for 30 seconds. Add beef, in batches, and cook, stirring, adding additional oil if necessary, until browned, about 4 minutes per batch. Transfer to slow cooker stoneware.

2. Reduce heat to medium. Add onions to pan and cook, stirring, until softened, about 3 minutes. Add garlic, gingerroot, peppercorns, cinnamon stick and bay leaf and cook, stirring, for 1 minute. Add broth and bring to a boil. Transfer to slow cooker stoneware.

NUTRIENTS PER SERVING	
Calories	235
Fat	8.5 g
Saturates	2.4 g
Polyunsaturates	0.8 g
Monounsaturates	3.9 g
Cholesterol	37 mg
Sodium	378 mg
Carbohydrate	18.3 g
Fiber	4.3 g
Protein	21.8 g

AMERICA'S EXCHANGES	
1	Starch
1	Vegetable
2½	Lean Meat

CANADA'S CHOICES	
1	Carbohydrate
2½	Meat and Alternatives

Make Ahead

This dish can be partially prepared before it is cooked. Heat 1 tbsp (15 mL) of the oil and complete Step 2. Cover and refrigerate overnight or for up to 2 days. When you're ready to cook, either brown the beef as outlined in Step 1 or add it to the stoneware without browning. Stir well and continue with Step 3.

3. Add chickpeas and stir well. Cover and cook on Low for 8 hours or on High for 4 hours, until beef is tender. Add curry powder solution and stir well. Add spinach, in batches, stirring, until each batch is submerged in the curry. Cover and cook on High for 20 minutes, until spinach is wilted. Discard cinnamon stick and bay leaf. Ladle into bowls and drizzle with yogurt, if using.

Mindful Morsels

Meat is one of the best food sources of vitamin B_{12}, which works in conjunction with other substances to help the body develop red blood cells and nerve cells, among other functions.

Tips

Substitute an equal quantity of lemon thyme for the thyme, if you prefer.

To toast cumin seeds: Place seeds in a skillet over medium heat, stirring, until fragrant and they just begin to brown, about 3 minutes. Immediately transfer to a mortar or spice grinder and grind.

This produces a mildly flavored stew. If you like the taste of cumin, feel free to increase the quantity to as much as 2 tbsp (25 mL).

If you don't have a mortar or a spice grinder, place the toasted cumin seeds on a cutting board and use the bottom of a wine bottle or measuring cup to grind them.

Canned tomatoes vary in sizes. If your supermarket carries the 19-oz (540 mL) can of diced tomatoes, by all means substitute it in this recipe.

For convenience, use bottled roasted red peppers if you don't have the time or inclination to roast your own.

Mediterranean Beef Ragout

Succulent peppers, sweet or hot, are so much a part of Mediterranean cooking that it's interesting to recall they are indigenous to North America and didn't cross the Atlantic until Columbus brought them to Spain. Here they combine with cumin, olives and tomatoes to transform humble stewing beef into an epicurean delight.

- **Works in slow cookers from 3½ to 6 quarts**

¼ cup	all-purpose flour	50 mL
1 tsp	dried thyme leaves, crumbled	5 mL
1 tsp	grated lemon zest, optional	5 mL
½ tsp	salt	2 mL
½ tsp	cracked black peppercorns	2 mL
2 lbs	trimmed stewing beef, cut into 1-inch (2.5 cm) cubes	1 kg
2 tbsp	olive oil, divided	25 mL
2	onions, chopped	2
4	cloves garlic, minced	4
1 tbsp	cumin seeds, toasted and ground (see Tips, left)	15 mL
1 cup	lower-salt beef broth	250 mL
½ cup	dry red wine	125 mL
1	can (14 oz/398 mL) diced tomatoes, including juice (see Tips, left)	1
2	bay leaves	2
2	roasted red bell peppers, thinly sliced, then cut into 1-inch (2.5 cm) pieces (see Tips, left)	2
½ cup	sliced pitted green olives	125 mL
½ cup	finely chopped parsley	125 mL

1. In a resealable plastic bag, combine flour, thyme, lemon zest, if using, salt and peppercorns. Add beef and toss until evenly coated. Set aside, shaking any excess flour from beef and reserving.

2. In a skillet, heat 1 tbsp (15 mL) of the oil over medium-high heat for 30 seconds. Add beef, in batches, and cook, stirring, adding more oil as necessary, until browned, about 4 minutes per batch. Transfer to slow cooker stoneware.

NUTRIENTS PER SERVING	
Calories	216
Fat	10.4 g
Saturates	2.9 g
Polyunsaturates	0.7 g
Monounsaturates	5.2 g
Cholesterol	44 mg
Sodium	542 mg
Carbohydrate	8.4 g
Fiber	1.3 g
Protein	21.9 g

AMERICA'S EXCHANGES	
1½	Vegetable
2½	Lean Meat
½	Fat

CANADA'S CHOICES	
½	Carbohydrate
3	Meat and Alternatives

Make Ahead

This dish can be partially prepared before it is cooked. Heat oil and complete Step 3. Refrigerate overnight or for up to 2 days. When you're ready to cook, complete Steps 1, 2 and 4.

3. Reduce heat to medium. Add onions and garlic to pan and cook, stirring, until onions are softened, about 3 minutes. Sprinkle with toasted cumin and flour mixture and cook, stirring, for 1 minute. Add broth, wine, tomatoes, with juice, and bay leaves and bring to a boil. Cook, stirring, until slightly thickened, about 2 minutes. Add to slow cooker and stir well.

4. Cover and cook on Low for 8 hours or on High for 4 hours, until mixture is bubbly and beef is tender. Stir in roasted peppers, olives and parsley. Cover and cook on High for 15 minutes, until peppers are heated through. Discard bay leaves.

Mindful Morsels

Like all animal foods, the meat in this recipe is a source of dietary cholesterol. The relationship between the cholesterol you consume in food and the cholesterol in your blood is not clear, although research shows that some people react more than others to the cholesterol in foods. However, the American Heart Association recommends that healthy adults consume less than 300 mg of dietary cholesterol a day.

Tips

I prefer to use sweet paprika in this recipe, but if you like a bit of heat, use hot paprika, instead, reducing the quantity to 2 tsp (10 mL).

One way of preparing collard greens for use in a stew is to cut them into a chiffonade. Remove any tough veins toward the bottom of the leaves and up the center of the lower portion of the leaf. Stack about 6 leaves in a pile. Roll them up like a cigar, then slice as thinly as you can. Repeat until all the greens are sliced.

Carbonnade with Collards

Carbonnade, a stew made of beef, onions and beer, is a favorite dish in Belgium. It is hearty bistro food, often flavored with bacon and brown sugar. Although it is great comfort food, carbonnade can be a tad bland and extremely rich. I prefer this lighter version with a hint of spice rather than sweetness, and the addition of flavorful and nutrient-dense collard greens. Serve this over hot whole wheat fettuccine, brown rice noodles or mashed potatoes for a meal that is destined to become a family favorite.

- **Works in slow cookers from 3½ to 6 quarts**

2 tbsp	olive oil, divided (approx.)	25 mL
2 lbs	trimmed stewing beef, cut into 1-inch (2.5 cm) cubes	1 kg
3	onions, thinly sliced on the vertical	3
4	cloves garlic, minced	4
1 tsp	dried thyme leaves, crumbled	5 mL
1 tsp	salt	5 mL
½ tsp	cracked black peppercorns	2 mL
2 tbsp	all-purpose flour	25 mL
1 tbsp	tomato paste	15 mL
2 cups	dark beer	500 mL
½ cup	lower-salt chicken broth	125 mL
2	bay leaves	2
1 tbsp	paprika, dissolved in 2 tbsp (25 mL) cider vinegar (see Tips, left)	15 mL
8 cups	thinly sliced (chiffonade) stemmed collard greens (about 2 bunches) (see Tips, left)	2 L

1. In a skillet, heat 1 tbsp (15 mL) of the oil over medium-high heat for 30 seconds. Add beef, in batches, and cook, stirring, adding more oil as necessary, until browned, about 5 minutes per batch. Transfer to slow cooker stoneware.

2. Reduce heat to medium. Add onions to pan and cook, stirring, until softened, about 3 minutes. Add garlic, thyme, salt and peppercorns and cook, stirring, for 1 minute. Add flour and cook, stirring, until lightly browned, about 2 minutes. Stir in tomato paste. Add beer, broth and bay leaves and bring to a boil. Cook, stirring, for 1 minute, scraping up all brown bits in the pan. Transfer to slow cooker stoneware. Stir well.

NUTRIENTS PER SERVING	
Calories	213
Fat	9.4 g
Saturates	2.7 g
Polyunsaturates	0.7 g
Monounsaturates	4.5 g
Cholesterol	44 mg
Sodium	326 mg
Carbohydrate	10.0 g
Fiber	1.8 g
Protein	21.8 g

AMERICA'S EXCHANGES	
2	Vegetable
3	Lean Meat

CANADA'S CHOICES	
½	Carbohydrate
3	Meat and Alternatives

Make Ahead

Heat 1 tbsp (15 mL) of the oil and complete Step 2. Cover and refrigerate overnight or for up to 2 days. When you're ready to cook, either brown the beef as outlined in Step 1 or add it to the stoneware without browning. Stir well and continue with Step 3.

3. Cover and cook on Low for 8 hours or on High for 4 hours, until meat is tender. Add paprika solution and stir well. Add collard greens, in batches, completely submerging each batch in the liquid before adding another. Cover and cook on High for 30 minutes, until collards are tender. Discard bay leaves.

Mindful Morsels

Like all meat, beef is a good source of zinc. Among its functions, zinc stimulates enzyme activity, helps wounds heal, boosts the immune system and supports growth during key periods of development. Poultry, fish, whole grains, legumes, nuts and seeds, particularly pumpkin seeds, also contain varying amounts of zinc.

Moroccan-Spiced Beef

Tip

To toast cumin and coriander seeds: Place seeds in a dry skillet over medium heat and toast, stirring, until fragrant and cumin seeds just begin to brown, about 3 minutes. Immediately transfer to a mortar or a spice grinder and grind.

Here's a stew that is every bit as delicious as it is unusual. I love the hint of sweetness provided by the parsnips and the way the cumin, coriander, cinnamon, black peppercorns and cayenne combine to create the richly flavored broth. Accompanied by a bowl of steaming couscous, this makes a perfect meal for any occasion.

- **Large (minimum 5 quart) slow cooker**

1 tbsp	olive oil	15 mL
2 lbs	trimmed stewing beef, cut into 1-inch (2.5 cm) cubes	1 kg
2	onions, chopped	2
4	large carrots, peeled and chopped (about 1 lb/500 g)	4
4	large parsnips, peeled and chopped (about 1 lb/500 g)	4
4	cloves garlic, minced	4
1 tsp	cracked black peppercorns	5 mL
1	piece (6 inches/15 cm) cinnamon stick	1
2 tbsp	cumin seeds, toasted and ground (see Tip, left)	25 mL
2 tsp	coriander seeds, toasted and ground	10 mL
2 tbsp	all-purpose flour	25 mL
1	can (28 oz/796 mL) diced tomatoes, drained	1
1 tbsp	tomato paste	15 mL
1 cup	lower-salt beef broth	250 mL
½ cup	dry red wine	125 mL
½ tsp	cayenne pepper	2 mL
1 tbsp	freshly squeezed lemon juice	15 mL
	Finely chopped parsley	

1. In a skillet, heat half the oil over medium-high heat for 30 seconds. Add beef, in batches, and cook, stirring, adding remaining oil as necessary, until lightly browned, about 4 minutes per batch. Using a slotted spoon, transfer to slow cooker stoneware.

2. Reduce heat to medium. Add onions, carrots and parsnips to pan and cook, stirring, until carrots are softened, about 7 minutes. Add garlic, peppercorns, cinnamon stick and toasted ground seeds and cook, stirring, for 1 minute. Add flour and cook, stirring, for 1 minute. Add tomatoes, tomato paste, broth and red wine and bring to a boil, stirring.

NUTRIENTS PER SERVING	
Calories	277
Fat	9.5 g
Saturates	2.8 g
Polyunsaturates	0.7 g
Monounsaturates	4.0 g
Cholesterol	47 mg
Sodium	344 mg
Carbohydrate	24.0 g
Fiber	4.4 g
Protein	24.6 g

AMERICA'S EXCHANGES	
2	Vegetable
1	Other Carbohydrate
3	Lean Meat

CANADA'S CHOICES	
1	Carbohydrate
3	Meat and Alternatives

Make Ahead

This dish can be partially prepared before it is cooked. Complete Step 2, heating 1 tbsp (15 mL) oil in pan before softening the vegetables. Cover and refrigerate mixture overnight. The next morning, brown beef (Step 1), or if you're pressed for time, omit this step and add meat directly to stoneware. Continue cooking as directed in Step 3. Alternatively, cook stew overnight, but do not add the parsley. Cover and refrigerate for the day. When you're ready to serve, bring to a boil in a Dutch oven and simmer for 10 minutes, until meat is heated through and sauce is bubbly. Stir in the parsley and serve.

3. Transfer to slow cooker stoneware. Cover and cook on Low for 8 hours or on High for 4 hours, until vegetables are tender. Dissolve cayenne in lemon juice and stir into mixture. Garnish liberally with parsley before serving. Serve with couscous.

Mindful Morsels

When one thinks about vegetables, parsnips are usually a bit of an afterthought, which is unfortunate. They belong to the same plant family as parsley, coriander, carrots and celery. A half-cup (125 mL) of cooked parsnips is high in folacin and potassium, and is a source of several other nutrients, including fiber, vitamin C and magnesium.

Tips

This quantity of black peppercorns provides a nicely zesty result. If you prefer a less peppery dish, reduce the quantity by half.

In my opinion, cauliflower needs to be cooked quickly in rapidly boiling water. Cook it until it's tender to the bite, about 3 minutes after the water has returned to a boil, drain and add to the slow cooker.

Serve this over long-grain brown rice, with a cucumber salad on the side.

Make Ahead

This dish can be partially prepared before it is cooked. Heat oil and complete Step 2. Cover and refrigerate overnight or for up to 2 days. When you're ready to cook, either brown the beef as outlined in Step 1 or add it to the stoneware without browning. Stir well and continue with Step 3.

Variation

Substitute 4 cups (1 L) broccoli florets for the cauliflower.

NUTRIENTS PER SERVING	
Calories	210
Fat	10.1 g
Saturates	2.7 g
Polyunsaturates	1.0 g
Monounsaturates	4.7 g
Cholesterol	44 mg
Sodium	167 mg
Carbohydrate	7.5 g
Fiber	2.7 g
Protein	22.9 g

Indian Beef with Cauliflower and Peppers

If you have a hankering for something that resembles a beef curry but is more nutritious, here's the recipe for you.

- **Works in slow cookers from 3½ to 6 quarts**

1 tbsp	olive oil (approx.)	15 mL
2 lbs	trimmed stewing beef, cut into ½-inch (1 cm) cubes	1 kg
2	onions, finely chopped	2
1 tbsp	minced gingerroot	15 mL
2	cloves garlic, minced	2
1	piece (2 inches/5 cm) cinnamon stick	1
1 tsp	cracked black peppercorns (see Tips, left)	5 mL
2	bay leaves	2
2 tbsp	cumin seeds, toasted and ground (see Tip, page 196)	25 mL
1 tbsp	coriander seeds, toasted and ground	15 mL
1 cup	lower-salt beef broth	250 mL
2 tbsp	tomato paste	25 mL
1	red bell pepper, diced	1
1 to 2	long green chile peppers, minced	1 to 2
4 cups	cooked cauliflower florets (see Tips, left)	1 L
	Low-fat plain yogurt	
¼ cup	toasted slivered almonds	50 mL
½ cup	finely chopped cilantro leaves	125 mL

1. In a skillet, heat half the oil over medium-high heat for 30 seconds. Add beef, in batches, and cook, stirring, adding remaining oil as necessary, until browned, about 4 minutes per batch. Using a slotted spoon, transfer to slow cooker stoneware.

2. Reduce heat to medium. Add onions to pan and cook, stirring, until softened, about 3 minutes. Add gingerroot, garlic, cinnamon stick, peppercorns, bay leaves, cumin and coriander and cook, stirring, for 1 minute. Add broth and tomato paste and bring to a boil, scraping up brown bits in the pan. Transfer to slow cooker stoneware. Stir well.

3. Cover and cook on Low for 6 to 8 hours or on High for 3 to 4 hours, until beef is tender. Discard bay leaves and cinnamon stick. Add red pepper and chile pepper and stir well. Stir in cooked cauliflower. Cover and cook on High for 20 minutes, until pepper is tender. To serve, garnish with a drizzle of yogurt, toasted almonds and cilantro.

AMERICA'S EXCHANGES	
1	Vegetable
3	Lean Meat

CANADA'S CHOICES	
3	Meat and Alternatives
1	Extra

MAKES 8 SERVINGS

Tips

This quantity of dried mushrooms equates to half of a ½-oz (14 g) package. Crumbling them with your fingers before soaking eliminates the need to chop them, and the powdery texture works well.

Although pearl barley is more readily available, make an effort to find whole (also known as hulled) barley when making the recipes in this book. It contains more nutrients, including fiber, than its refined relative. Pot barley, which is more refined than whole barley, is also a preferable alternative to pearl barley as it maintains some of the bran.

Make Ahead

This dish can be partially prepared before it is cooked. Complete Steps 1 and 2. Cover and refrigerate overnight. The next morning, continue with the recipe.

NUTRIENTS PER SERVING	
Calories	261
Fat	10.3 g
Saturates	3.5 g
Polyunsaturates	0.7 g
Monounsaturates	4.9 g
Cholesterol	34 mg
Sodium	421 mg
Carbohydrate	28.1 g
Fiber	3.6 g
Protein	15.3 g

Beef Collops with Barley

"Collops" is a Scottish term for a dish made from scallops of meat or minced meat, stewed with onion and a sauce. I've updated this version to include dried mushrooms for enhanced flavor and have added barley for nutrition, transforming it into a casserole. With its flavorful gravy and soothing grain base, this is the ultimate comfort food dish and is perfect for those evenings when everyone is coming and going at different times. Just leave it in the slow cooker on Warm and people can help themselves. Leave the fixin's for salad and whole grain rolls to complete the meal.

• **Large (minimum 5 quart) slow cooker**

2 tbsp	dried wild mushrooms, crumbled (see Tips, left)	25 mL
½ cup	hot water	125 mL
1 tbsp	olive oil	15 mL
1 lb	lean ground beef	500 g
2	onions, finely chopped	2
4	cloves garlic, minced	4
1 tbsp	fresh rosemary leaves, finely chopped, or 2 tsp (10 mL) dried rosemary, crumbled	15 mL
½ tsp	cracked black peppercorns	2 mL
12 oz	cremini mushrooms, sliced	375 g
1	can (28 oz/796 mL) diced tomatoes, drained	1
2 cups	lower-salt beef broth	500 mL
1 cup	barley, rinsed (see Tips, left)	250 mL

1. In a heatproof bowl, combine dried mushrooms and hot water. Stir well and let stand for 30 minutes. Strain through a fine sieve, reserving mushrooms and liquid separately. Set aside.

2. In a skillet, heat oil over medium heat for 30 seconds. Add beef and onions and cook, stirring and breaking beef up with a spoon, until beef is no longer pink, about 5 minutes. Add garlic, rosemary, peppercorns and reserved soaked mushrooms and cook, stirring, for 1 minute. Add cremini mushrooms and stir well. Add tomatoes, broth and reserved mushroom liquid and bring to a boil.

3. Transfer to slow cooker stoneware. Stir in barley. Cover and cook on Low for 6 to 8 hours or on High for 3 to 4 hours, until barley is tender.

AMERICA'S EXCHANGES	
1½	Starch
1	Vegetable
1½	Medium-fat Meat
½	Fat

CANADA'S CHOICES	
1½	Carbohydrate
1½	Meat and Alternatives
½	Fat

Tip

Chile nomenclature can be confusing. Long red or green chiles are usually used in Indian cooking and can be found in Asian markets. They are sometimes called cayenne or serrano chiles, not to be confused with Mexican serrano chiles, which are different.

Make Ahead

This dish can be partially prepared before it is cooked. Complete Step 2, heating 1 tbsp (15 mL) oil in pan before softening onions. Cover and refrigerate for up to 2 days. When you're ready to cook, brown beef (Step 1), or omit this step and place meat directly in stoneware. Continue cooking as directed in Step 3.

Braised Beef Curry with Fragrant Spices

In this Indian-inspired dish, chunks of beef cook in their own juices, seasoned with spices. Using whole spices such as cloves and coriander seeds and cinnamon sticks, rather than ground versions, improves the result since they release their flavor slowly as the curry cooks. Serve with lots of fluffy white rice and Indian bread such as naan to soak up the delicious sauce.

• **Works in slow cookers from 3½ to 5 quarts**

1 tbsp	olive oil	15 mL
2 lbs	trimmed stewing beef, cut into 1-inch (2.5 cm) cubes	1 kg
2	onions, finely chopped	2
4	cloves garlic, minced	4
1 tbsp	minced gingerroot	15 mL
1 tbsp	coriander seeds	15 mL
1 tsp	turmeric	5 mL
1	piece (2 inches/5 cm) cinnamon stick	1
4	whole cloves	4
1 tsp	salt	5 mL
1 tsp	cracked black peppercorns	5 mL
½ tsp	fennel seeds	2 mL
¼ cup	lower-salt beef broth	50 mL
2	long red or green chiles, finely chopped (see Tip, left)	2

1. In a skillet, heat half the oil over medium-high heat for 30 seconds. Add beef, in batches, and cook, stirring, adding remaining oil as necessary, until nicely browned, about 4 minutes per batch. Using a slotted spoon, transfer to slow cooker stoneware.

2. Reduce heat to medium. Add onions to pan and cook, stirring, until softened, about 3 minutes. Add garlic, gingerroot, coriander seeds, turmeric, cinnamon stick, cloves, salt, peppercorns and fennel seeds and cook, stirring, for 1 minute. Add broth and bring to a boil.

3. Pour mixture over beef. Cover and cook on Low for 8 to 10 hours or on High for 4 to 5 hours, until beef is tender. Stir in chiles. Cover and cook on High for 10 minutes. Serve immediately.

NUTRIENTS PER SERVING	
Calories	190
Fat	8.8 g
Saturates	2.7 g
Polyunsaturates	0.5 g
Monounsaturates	4.0 g
Cholesterol	47 mg
Sodium	387 mg
Carbohydrate	4.8 g
Fiber	1.0 g
Protein	22.2 g

AMERICA'S EXCHANGES	
1	Vegetable
3	Lean Meat

CANADA'S CHOICES	
3	Meat and Alternatives

Tips

Canned tomatoes vary in sizes. If your supermarket carries the 19-oz (540 mL) can of diced tomatoes, by all means substitute it in this recipe.

Use an apple corer to make the cavities for stuffing.

Make Ahead

This dish can be assembled before it is cooked. Complete Steps 1 through 3. Cool filling thoroughly, then continue with Step 4. Cover and refrigerate overnight or for up to 2 days. When you're ready to cook, continue with Step 5.

Stuffed Onions

Here's a tasty solution to the midweek dining blues — ground-beef-and-bulgur-filled onions, topped with Parmesan and dill. Use any sweet onion — Vidalia, Spanish and red onions all work well. Just make sure they are as crisp and fresh as possible and that all will fit in the stoneware. Serve these with a tossed green salad, sprinkled with shredded carrots to add a sparkle of color along with nutrients and flavor.

- **Large (minimum 6 quart) oval slow cooker**

½ cup	bulgur	125 mL
½ cup	boiling water	125 mL
6	large sweet onions	6
1 tbsp	olive oil	15 mL
12 oz	extra-lean ground beef	375 g
6	cloves garlic, minced	6
1 tsp	dried oregano leaves, crumbled	5 mL
½ tsp	salt	2 mL
½ tsp	cracked black peppercorns	2 mL
½ cup	dry white wine or lower-salt chicken broth	125 mL
1	can (14 oz/398 mL) diced tomatoes, including juice (see Tips, page left)	1
½ cup	grated Parmesan cheese	125 mL
½ cup	finely chopped dill or parsley	125 mL

1. In a bowl, combine bulgur and boiling water. Set aside for 20 minutes.

2. Cut off tops and bottoms of onions and peel. Hollow out the centers (see Tip, left) and discard. Drop prepared onions into a large pot of boiling water and blanch for 5 minutes. Drain and rinse in cold water. Place in slow cooker stoneware with the hollows pointing up.

3. In a skillet, heat oil over medium heat for 30 seconds. Add ground beef, garlic, oregano, salt and peppercorns and cook, stirring and breaking up with a spoon, until meat is no longer pink, about 5 minutes. Add white wine and tomatoes with juice and bring to a boil. Stir in bulgur.

4. Fill centers of onions with beef mixture, using a blunt object such as a kitchen knife to pack the filling in as tightly as possible. Pour remaining filling over onions.

5. Cover and cook on Low for 8 hours or on High for 4 hours, until onions are tender and mixture is hot and bubbly. To serve, place an onion on each plate. Sprinkle with Parmesan and garnish with dill.

NUTRIENTS PER SERVING	
Calories	294
Fat	9.6 g
Saturates	3.7 g
Polyunsaturates	0.5 g
Monounsaturates	4.3 g
Cholesterol	38 mg
Sodium	508 mg
Carbohydrate	34.2 g
Fiber	4.4 g
Protein	19.8 g

AMERICA'S EXCHANGES	
1	Starch
1½	Carbohydrate
2	Medium-fat Meat

CANADA'S CHOICES	
2	Carbohydrate
2	Meat and Alternatives

Tip

Buckwheat groats are also known as kasha. If you prefer, you may substitute an equal quantity of bulgur. If using bulgur, combine it with the boiling water and set aside until all the water is absorbed, about 20 minutes. Continue with Step 2.

Buckwheat Meatballs in Tomato Sauce

More like a saucy meatloaf than traditional meatballs swimming in sauce, this tasty dish is as much at home over hot cooked rice or fluffy mashed potatoes as it is over pasta. I like to serve this with a platter of steamed bitter greens, such as rapini, drizzled with extra virgin olive oil and freshly squeezed lemon juice, but steamed broccoli also makes a nice accompaniment.

- **Works in slow cookers from 3½ to 6 quarts**

Meatballs

½ cup	buckwheat groats (see Tips, left)	125 mL
1 cup	boiling water	250 mL
1	onion, finely chopped	1
½ cup	finely chopped parsley	125 mL
½ tsp	salt	2 mL
¼ tsp	freshly ground black pepper	1 mL
¼ tsp	ground cinnamon	1 mL
1 lb	lean ground beef	500 g
1	egg, beaten	1
2 tbsp	olive oil (approx.), divided	25 mL

Tomato Sauce

2	onions, finely chopped	2
4	cloves garlic, minced	4
1 tsp	dried oregano leaves, crumbled	5 mL
½ tsp	salt	2 mL
½ tsp	cracked black peppercorns	2 mL
1	can (28 oz/796 mL) diced tomatoes, including juice	1
1 cup	dry red wine	250 mL

1. **Meatballs:** In a saucepan, combine buckwheat groats and boiling water. Cover and cook over low heat until all the water has been absorbed, about 20 minutes. Remove from heat and set aside.

2. In a bowl, mix together onion, parsley, salt, pepper and cinnamon. Add ground beef and egg, and using your hands, mix until well combined. Using a wooden spoon (it will still be hot), mix in cooked buckwheat. Form into 24 meatballs, each about 1½ inches (4 cm) in diameter.

NUTRIENTS PER SERVING	
Calories	233
Fat	12.2 g
Saturates	3.8 g
Polyunsaturates	0.7 g
Monounsaturates	6.3 g
Cholesterol	57 mg
Sodium	484 mg
Carbohydrate	17.1 g
Fiber	2.7 g
Protein	14.9 g

AMERICA'S EXCHANGES	
½	Starch
2	Vegetable
2	Medium-fat Meat

CANADA'S CHOICES	
1	Carbohydrate
2	Meat and Alternatives
½	Fat

Do all your preparation for the sauce as well as the meatballs while the kasha cooks so you'll be ready to start cooking as soon as it is completed.

3. In a skillet, heat 1 tbsp (15 mL) of the oil over medium-high heat. Add meatballs, in batches, and brown well, about 5 minutes per batch. Transfer to slow cooker stoneware.

4. **Tomato Sauce:** Reduce heat to medium and add additional oil if necessary. Add onions to pan and cook, stirring, until softened, about 3 minutes. Add garlic, oregano, salt and peppercorns and cook, stirring, for 1 minute. Add tomatoes, with juice, and wine and bring to a boil.

5. Pour over meatballs. Cover and cook on Low for 7 hours or on High for $3\frac{1}{2}$ hours, until hot and bubbly.

Mindful Morsels

Despite its name, buckwheat is not a form of wheat and does not contain gluten, making it an ideal "grain" for people with gluten sensitivity. In fact, buckwheat is technically a fruit.

Tips

Pre-packaged veal shank slices are usually too big for a single serving of this recipe. Ask the butcher to cut the veal shank into 1-inch (2.5 cm) slices.

To clean leeks: Fill a sink full of lukewarm water. Split the leeks in half lengthwise and submerge them in the water, swishing them around to remove all traces of dirt. Transfer to a colander and rinse thoroughly under cold water.

Osso Buco with Lemon Gremolata

This is probably my all-time favorite veal dish. I love the wine-flavored sauce and the succulent meat, enhanced with just a soupçon of gremolata, pungent with fresh garlic and lemon zest. But best of all, I adore eating the marrow from the bones, a rare and delicious treat. Pass coffee spoons to ensure that every mouthwatering morsel is extracted from the bone.

- **Large (minimum 5 quart) slow cooker**

1	package (½ oz/14 g) dried porcini mushrooms	1
1 cup	boiling water	250 mL
¼ cup	all-purpose flour	50 mL
1 tsp	salt	5 mL
½ tsp	freshly ground black pepper	2 mL
8	sliced veal shanks (each about 6 oz/170 g) (see Tips, left)	8
1 tbsp	olive oil	15 mL
1 tbsp	butter	15 mL
3	leeks, white part only, cleaned and thinly sliced (see Tips, left)	3
2	carrots, peeled and finely chopped	2
2	stalks celery, finely chopped	2
2	cloves garlic, finely chopped	2
1 tsp	dried thyme or 2 sprigs fresh thyme	5 mL
½ cup	dry white wine	125 mL

Lemon Gremolata

2	cloves garlic, minced	2
1 cup	finely chopped parsley	250 mL
	Grated zest of 1 lemon	
1 tbsp	extra virgin olive oil	15 mL

1. In a heatproof bowl, combine porcini mushrooms and boiling water. Let stand for 30 minutes. Drain through a fine sieve, reserving liquid. Pat mushrooms dry with paper towel and chop finely. Set aside.

2. In a bowl, mix together flour, salt and black pepper. Lightly coat veal shanks with mixture, shaking off the excess. Set any flour mixture remaining aside.

3. In a large skillet, heat olive oil and butter over medium heat. Add veal and cook until lightly browned on both sides. Transfer to slow cooker stoneware.

NUTRIENTS PER SERVING	
Calories	205
Fat	6.7 g
Saturates	2.1 g
Polyunsaturates	0.6 g
Monounsaturates	2.9 g
Cholesterol	101 mg
Sodium	390 mg
Carbohydrate	11.7 g
Fiber	2.5 g
Protein	23.9 g

AMERICA'S EXCHANGES	
1½	Vegetable
3	Lean Meat

CANADA'S CHOICES	
½	Carbohydrate
3	Meat and Alternatives

Make Ahead

This dish can be partially prepared before it is cooked. Complete Steps 1 and 4, heating 1 tbsp (15 mL) olive oil in pan before softening leeks, carrots and celery. Cover sauce and refrigerate for up to 2 days. When you're ready to cook, continue with the recipe. Alternatively, Osso Buco can be cooked overnight in slow cooker, covered and refrigerated for up to 2 days. When ready to serve, spoon off congealed fat and transfer stew to a Dutch oven. Bring to a boil and simmer for 10 minutes, until meat is heated through and sauce is bubbly.

4. Add leeks, carrots and celery to pan and stir well. Reduce heat to low, cover and cook until vegetables are softened, about 10 minutes. Increase heat to medium. Add garlic, thyme and reserved mushrooms and cook, stirring, for 1 minute. Add reserved flour mixture, and cook, stirring, for 1 minute. Add wine and reserved mushroom liquid and bring to a boil.

5. Pour mixture over veal, cover and cook on Low for 12 hours, until veal is very tender.

6. **Lemon Gremolata:** Just before serving, combine garlic, parsley, lemon zest and olive oil in a small serving bowl and pass around the table, allowing guests to individually garnish.

Mindful Morsels

The dried porcini mushrooms in this recipe add deep and delicious flavor to the luscious sauce. Not only are mushrooms very low in calories (less than 20 calories per cup/250 mL raw sliced), but they are also a source of potassium, which helps control blood pressure, and zinc, which helps your immune system function.

Tip

If you are using fresh rosemary and prefer a more pronounced flavor, bury a whole sprig in the meat before adding the sauce. Remove before serving.

Make Ahead

This dish can be partially prepared before it is cooked. Complete Steps 1 and 3, refrigerating mixture for up to 2 days. When you're ready to cook, place veal in slow cooker (don't bother with browning) and continue with Step 4.

Wine-Braised Veal with Rosemary

This is a delicious Italian-inspired stew that is both simple and elegant. Serve over hot Basic Polenta (see recipe, page 229) and accompany with steamed broccoli or rapini.

- **Large (minimum 5 quart) slow cooker**

3	slices bacon, cut crosswise into thin strips	3
1 tbsp	olive oil	15 mL
2 lbs	trimmed stewing veal, cut into 1-inch (2.5 cm) cubes	1 kg
3	leeks, white part only, cleaned and coarsely chopped	3
3	large carrots, peeled and diced	3
2	stalks celery, diced	2
2	cloves garlic, minced	2
1½ tbsp	chopped fresh rosemary leaves or dried rosemary leaves, crumbled (see Tip, left)	22 mL
1 tsp	salt	5 mL
½ tsp	cracked black peppercorns	2 mL
2 tbsp	all-purpose flour	25 mL
½ cup	dry red wine	125 mL
½ cup	lower-salt chicken broth	125 mL
	Fresh rosemary sprigs, optional	

1. Heat a skillet over medium heat for 30 seconds. Add bacon and cook, stirring, until crisp. Drain off fat.

2. Add half the oil. Add the veal, in batches, and cook, stirring, adding remaining oil as necessary, just until it begins to brown, about 4 minutes. Using a slotted spoon, transfer to slow cooker stoneware.

3. Add leeks, carrots and celery to pan and cook, stirring, until softened, about 7 minutes. Add garlic, rosemary, salt, peppercorns and reserved bacon and cook, stirring, for 1 minute. Sprinkle flour over mixture and cook, stirring, for 1 minute. Add wine and broth and cook, stirring, until mixture thickens.

4. Pour mixture over meat and stir to combine. Cover and cook on Low for 8 to 10 hours or on High for 4 to 6 hours, until meat is tender. Garnish with rosemary sprigs, if using, and serve.

NUTRIENTS PER SERVING	
Calories	158
Fat	4.8 g
Saturates	1.2 g
Polyunsaturates	0.6 g
Monounsaturates	2.2 g
Cholesterol	78 mg
Sodium	388 mg
Carbohydrate	8.2 g
Fiber	2.1 g
Protein	20.0 g

AMERICA'S EXCHANGES	
1½	Vegetable
2½	Lean Meat

CANADA'S CHOICES	
½	Carbohydrate
2½	Meat and Alternatives

Make Ahead

This dish can be partially prepared before it is cooked. Complete Step 3. Cover and refrigerate for up to 2 days. When you're ready to cook, continue with the recipe.

Dilled Veal Stew

This is a streamlined and lower-fat version of a Veal Blanquette I've been making for many years from The Silver Palate Cookbook. *I like to serve this for Sunday dinner, over hot whole wheat fettuccine or brown rice noodles.*

- **Large (minimum 5 quart) slow cooker**

2 tbsp	all-purpose flour	25 mL
1 tbsp	paprika	15 mL
¼ tsp	ground nutmeg	1 mL
1 tsp	salt	5 mL
½ tsp	freshly ground black pepper	2 mL
1 tbsp	butter	15 mL
2 tbsp	olive oil, divided	25 mL
2 lbs	trimmed stewing veal, cut into 1-inch (2.5 cm) cubes	1 kg
2	onions, thinly sliced	2
2	large carrots, peeled, cut into quarters lengthwise and very thinly sliced	2
4	stalks celery, thinly sliced	4
1 cup	lower-salt chicken broth	250 mL
½ cup	dry vermouth or white wine	125 mL
½ cup	whipping (35%) cream	125 mL
½ cup	finely chopped dill	125 mL
	Hot buttered noodles, optional	

1. In a bowl, combine flour, paprika, nutmeg, salt and pepper. Set aside.

2. In a skillet, melt butter and 1 tbsp (15 mL) of the oil over medium heat. Add veal and cook, stirring, for 3 to 4 minutes without browning. Sprinkle flour mixture over meat, stir to combine and, using a slotted spoon, transfer to slow cooker stoneware.

3. Add remaining oil to pan. Add onions, carrots and celery and cook, stirring, until vegetables are softened, about 7 minutes. Add broth and dry vermouth and bring to a boil.

4. Pour mixture over veal, cover and cook on Low for 8 to 10 hours or on High for 4 to 5 hours, until stew is hot and bubbly. Stir in cream and dill and serve over noodles, if desired.

NUTRIENTS PER SERVING	
Calories	204
Fat	10.7 g
Saturates	3.9 g
Polyunsaturates	0.8 g
Monounsaturates	5.0 g
Cholesterol	92 mg
Sodium	385 mg
Carbohydrate	6.4 g
Fiber	1.2 g
Protein	19.7 g

AMERICA'S EXCHANGES	
1	Vegetable
2½	Medium-fat Meat

CANADA'S CHOICES	
½	Carbohydrate
2½	Meat and Alternatives

Tips

There is a hint of caraway flavor in this version. If you prefer a stronger caraway flavor, increase the quantity of caraway seeds to as much as 2 tsp (10 mL).

I like to use small whole cremini mushrooms in this stew, but if you can't find them, white mushrooms or larger cremini mushrooms, quartered or sliced, depending upon their size, work well too.

Canned tomatoes vary in sizes. If your supermarket carries the 19-oz (540 mL) can of diced tomatoes, by all means substitute it in this recipe.

Veal Goulash

This version of goulash, a luscious Hungarian stew seasoned with paprika, is lighter than the traditional version made with beef. It is usually served over hot noodles, but fluffy mashed potatoes also make a sybaritic finish. The red bell peppers not only enhance the flavor, but also add valuable nutrients to the dish.

- **Works in slow cookers from 3¹⁄₂ to 6 quarts**

2 tbsp	olive oil, divided	25 mL
2 lbs	trimmed stewing veal, cut into 1-inch (2.5 cm) cubes	1 kg
2	onions, finely chopped	2
4	cloves garlic, minced	4
1 tsp	caraway seeds (see Tips, left)	5 mL
¹⁄₂ tsp	cracked black peppercorns	2 mL
1 lb	mushrooms (see Tips, left)	500 g
2 tbsp	all-purpose flour	25 mL
1	can (14 oz/398 mL) diced tomatoes, including juice (see Tips, page left)	1
1 cup	lower-salt chicken broth	250 mL
1 tbsp	sweet Hungarian paprika, dissolved in 2 tbsp (25 mL) water or lower-salt chicken broth	15 mL
2	red bell peppers, diced	2
¹⁄₂ cup	finely chopped dill	125 mL
	Sour cream, optional	

1. In a skillet, heat 1 tbsp (15 mL) of the oil over medium-high heat for 30 seconds. Add veal, in batches, and cook, stirring, adding more oil as necessary, until browned, about 5 minutes per batch. Using a slotted spoon, transfer to slow cooker stoneware.

2. Reduce heat to medium. Add onions to pan and cook, stirring, until softened, about 3 minutes. Add garlic, caraway seeds and peppercorns and cook, stirring, for 1 minute. Add mushrooms and toss to coat. Add flour and cook, stirring, for 1 minute. Add tomatoes, with juice, and broth and bring to a boil. Transfer to slow cooker stoneware. Stir well.

3. Cover and cook on Low for 8 hours or on High for 4 hours, until veal is tender.

NUTRIENTS PER SERVING	
Calories	207
Fat	6.8 g
Saturates	1.4 g
Polyunsaturates	0.8 g
Monounsaturates	3.5 g
Cholesterol	95 mg
Sodium	221 mg
Carbohydrate	11.3 g
Fiber	2.4 g
Protein	25.5 g

AMERICA'S EXCHANGES	
2	Vegetable
3	Lean Meat

CANADA'S CHOICES	
¹⁄₂	Carbohydrate
3	Meat and Alternatives

Make Ahead

This dish can be partially prepared before it is cooked. Heat 1 tbsp (15 mL) of the oil and complete Step 2. Cover and refrigerate overnight or for up to 1 day. When you're ready to cook, either brown the veal as outlined in Step 1 or add it to the stoneware without browning. Stir well and continue with Steps 3 and 4.

4. Add paprika solution to slow cooker stoneware and stir well. Add red peppers and stir well. Cover and cook on High for 30 minutes, until peppers are tender. To serve, ladle into bowls and top each serving with 1 tbsp (15 mL) of the dill and a dollop of sour cream, if using.

Mindful Morsels

Earthy and pungent, caraway is an ancient herb that has been used for medicinal and culinary purposes throughout history. It was used for centuries as a digestive aid and is often used to add balance to robust spice blends such as the fiery Tunisian harissa or the slightly sweet garam masala, which is used in Indian cooking. According to spice guru Ian Hemphill, Holland is the world's largest producer of caraway, and Dutch caraway seed is the world's best.

MAKES 6 SERVINGS

Tips

Pre-packaged veal shank slices are usually too big for a single serving of this recipe. Ask the butcher to cut the veal shank into 1-inch (2.5 cm) slices.

To clean leeks: Fill a sink full of lukewarm water. Split the leeks in half lengthwise and submerge them in the water, swishing them around to remove all traces of dirt. Transfer to a colander and rinse thoroughly under cold water.

Greek-Style Veal Shanks with Feta and Caper Gremolata

Although I love osso buco, an Italian method for preparing veal shanks, from time to time I pine for a different approach to this succulent cut of meat. This version puts a Greek spin on the dish with flavorings of garlic, oregano, white wine and a gremolata enhanced with feta and capers. Serve this over brown rice or hot orzo tossed with extra virgin olive oil, and add a platter of bitter greens, such as rapini, to complete the meal.

- **Works in slow cookers from 3½ to 6 quarts**

8	sliced veal shanks (each about 6 oz/170 g) (see Tips, left)	8
⅓ cup	all-purpose flour	75 mL
2 tbsp	olive oil, divided	25 mL
3	leeks, white part only, cleaned and thinly sliced (see Tips, left)	3
12	cloves garlic, slivered	12
2 tsp	dried oregano leaves, crumbled	10 mL
½ tsp	cracked black peppercorns	2 mL
1 cup	dry white wine	250 mL
3 tbsp	tomato paste	45 mL
2 cups	lower-salt chicken broth	500 mL

Gremolata

½ cup	finely chopped parsley	125 mL
1 tbsp	drained capers, minced	15 mL
1 tbsp	finely grated lemon zest	15 mL
¼ cup	crumbled feta	50 mL

1. On a plate, coat veal shanks with flour, shaking off excess. In a skillet, heat 1 tbsp (15 mL) of the oil over medium-high heat. Add veal, in batches, and cook, stirring, adding more oil as necessary, until lightly browned on all sides, about 5 minutes per batch. Transfer to slow cooker stoneware.

NUTRIENTS PER SERVING	
Calories	263
Fat	9.3 g
Saturates	2.3 g
Polyunsaturates	0.9 g
Monounsaturates	4.6 g
Cholesterol	100 mg
Sodium	365 mg
Carbohydrate	17.9 g
Fiber	3.6 g
Protein	26.9 g

AMERICA'S EXCHANGES	
1	Starch
1	Vegetable
3	Very Lean Meat
1	Fat

CANADA'S CHOICES	
1	Carbohydrate
3	Meat and Alternatives

Make Ahead

This dish can be partially prepared before it is cooked. Heat 1 tbsp (15 mL) of the oil and complete Step 2. Cover and refrigerate overnight or for up to 1 day. When you're ready to cook, complete Steps 1, 3 and 4.

2. Reduce heat to medium. Add leeks and cook, stirring, until softened, about 5 minutes. Add garlic, oregano and peppercorns and cook, stirring, for 1 minute. Add wine, tomato paste and broth, stirring, and bring to a boil. Transfer to slow cooker stoneware.

3. Cover and cook on Low for 12 hours or on High for 6 hours, until veal is very tender.

4. **Gremolata:** In a bowl, mix together parsley, capers and lemon zest. Add feta and stir until well integrated. Serve alongside veal.

Mindful Morsels

One serving of this dish provides a panoply of nutrients. It is an excellent source of vitamins B_6, B_{12} and K and the minerals phosphorus, potassium, iron and zinc. It is a good source of magnesium and folacin and a source of vitamins A and C and the mineral calcium. It also contains a moderate amount of dietary fiber.

Tip

A whole lamb shank is too big for a single serving of this recipe. Ask your butcher to cut each shank into two equal pieces.

Lamb Shanks with Luscious Legumes

Lamb cooked with legumes in a flavorful wine-based sauce is a French tradition. No wonder — it is a mouthwatering combination. If you prefer more assertive flavors, bury a whole branch of fresh rosemary, stem and all, in the lamb before adding the sauce. Serve this with crusty bread, a green salad or garden-fresh tomatoes in vinaigrette and a robust red wine for a memorable meal.

- **Works best in a large (minimum 5 quart) slow cooker**

2 cups	dried white navy beans or flageolets, soaked, rinsed and drained	500 mL
¼ cup	all-purpose flour	50 mL
1 tsp	salt	5 mL
½ tsp	cracked black peppercorns	2 mL
6	lamb shanks, sliced in half	6
2 tbsp	olive oil, divided	25 mL
2	onions, finely chopped	2
2	carrots, peeled and diced	2
4	stalks celery, diced	4
6	cloves garlic, minced	6
1 tbsp	finely chopped rosemary	15 mL
	Grated zest and juice of 1 orange	
1 cup	lower-salt beef broth	250 mL
½ cup	dry red wine	125 mL
	Finely chopped fresh parsley	

1. Place beans in slow cooker stoneware.

2. On a plate, combine flour, salt and peppercorns. Lightly coat lamb shanks with mixture, shaking off the excess. Set any remaining flour mixture aside.

3. In a skillet, heat 1 tbsp (15 mL) oil over medium-high heat. Add lamb, in batches, and cook, turning, adding more oil as necessary, until lightly browned on all sides. Using tongs, transfer to slow cooker stoneware. Drain all but 1 tbsp (15 mL) oil from pan.

NUTRIENTS PER SERVING	
Calories	253
Fat	6.5 g
Saturates	2.1 g
Polyunsaturates	0.7 g
Monounsaturates	3.2 g
Cholesterol	44 mg
Sodium	326 mg
Carbohydrate	27.7 g
Fiber	6.4 g
Protein	21.1 g

AMERICA'S EXCHANGES	
2	Starch
2½	Very Lean Meat

CANADA'S CHOICES	
1½	Carbohydrate
3	Meat and Alternatives

Make Ahead

This dish can be partially prepared before it is cooked. Soak beans. Complete Step 4, heating 1 tbsp (15 mL) of the oil in pan before softening vegetables and sprinkling 1 tbsp (15 mL) of the flour over the vegetables. Cover and refrigerate for up to 2 days. When you're ready to cook, continue with the recipe.

4. Reduce heat to medium. Add onions, carrots and celery to pan and cook, stirring, until carrots are softened, about 7 minutes. Add garlic, rosemary and orange zest and cook, stirring, for 1 minute. Sprinkle reserved flour mixture over vegetables and cook, stirring, for 1 minute. Add orange juice, broth and wine and bring to a boil.

5. Pour mixture over lamb. Cover and cook on Low for 10 to 12 hours or on High for 5 to 6 hours, until lamb is falling off the bone and beans are tender. Discard bones and transfer lamb and beans to a deep platter or serving dish; keep warm. In a saucepan over medium-high heat, reduce cooking liquid by one-third. Pour over lamb and garnish liberally with parsley.

Mindful Morsels

The navy beans in this recipe make it very high in fiber (over 6 g per serving).

This recipe can be partially prepared before it is cooked. Complete Step 3, heating 1 tbsp (15 mL) of the oil in pan before softening vegetables. Cover and refrigerate for up to 2 days. When you're ready to cook, brown lamb (Steps 1 and 2) and complete Step 4.

Irish Stew

This hearty and delicious stew is an old favorite that really can't be improved upon. All it needs is a green vegetable such as string beans or broccoli, a crusty roll and a glass of Guinness or a robust red wine.

- **Works best in a large (minimum 5 quart) slow cooker**

¼ cup	all-purpose flour	50 mL
1 tsp	salt	5 mL
½ tsp	cracked black peppercorns	2 mL
2 tbsp	olive oil, divided	25 mL
2 lbs	trimmed stewing lamb, cut into 1-inch (2.5 cm) cubes	1 kg
3	onions, finely chopped	3
2	large carrots, peeled and diced	2
1 tsp	dried thyme leaves	5 mL
2 tbsp	tomato paste	25 mL
1 tbsp	Worcestershire sauce	15 mL
1 cup	lower-salt beef broth	250 mL
4	medium potatoes, peeled and cut into ½-inch (1 cm) cubes	4
1½ cups	green peas	375 mL

1. On a plate, combine flour, salt and peppercorns. Lightly coat lamb with mixture, shaking off the excess. Set any remaining flour mixture aside.

2. In a skillet, heat 1 tbsp (15 mL) of the oil over medium-high heat for 30 seconds. Add lamb, in batches, and cook, stirring, adding more oil as necessary, until browned, about 4 minutes per batch. Using a slotted spoon, transfer to slow cooker stoneware. Drain all but 1 tbsp (15 mL) fat from pan.

3. Reduce heat to medium. Add onions and carrots to pan and cook, stirring, until carrots are softened, about 7 minutes. Add thyme and reserved flour mixture and cook, stirring, for 1 minute. Stir in tomato paste, Worcestershire sauce and broth and bring to a boil.

4. Place potatoes in slow cooker stoneware. Add onion mixture and stir to combine. Cover and cook on Low for 8 to 10 hours or on High for 4 to 5 hours, until mixture is bubbly and potatoes are tender. Stir in peas. Cover and cook on High for 15 to 20 minutes, until peas are heated through.

NUTRIENTS PER SERVING	
Calories	286
Fat	9.7 g
Saturates	2.7 g
Polyunsaturates	1.0 g
Monounsaturates	5.0 g
Cholesterol	73 mg
Sodium	567 mg
Carbohydrate	22.3 g
Fiber	3.2 g
Protein	26.8 g

AMERICA'S EXCHANGES	
1	Starch
1	Vegetable
3	Lean Meat

CANADA'S CHOICES	
1	Carbohydrate
3	Meat and Alternatives

Tips

If you can't find Swiss chard, use 2 packages (each 10 oz/300 g) fresh or frozen spinach. If using fresh spinach, remove the stems and chop leaves before using. If it has not been pre-washed, rinse it thoroughly in a basin of lukewarm water. If using frozen spinach, thaw it first.

Although this makes a large quantity, don't worry about leftovers. It reheats very well and may even be better the day after it is made.

Make Ahead

This dish can be partially prepared before it is cooked. Heat 1 tbsp (15 mL) of the oil and complete Step 2. Cover and refrigerate overnight or for up to 1 day. When you're ready to cook, either brown the lamb as outlined in Step 1 or add it to the stoneware without browning. Stir well and continue with Step 3.

NUTRIENTS PER SERVING	
Calories	277
Fat	6.8 g
Saturates	1.8 g
Polyunsaturates	0.8 g
Monounsaturates	3.3 g
Cholesterol	0 mg
Sodium	462 mg
Carbohydrate	29.6 g
Fiber	6.6 g
Protein	25.4 g

Lamb with Lentils and Chard

Rich with the flavors of the French countryside, this hearty stew is perfect for guests or a family meal. All it needs is a simple green salad, finished with a scattering of shredded carrots.

- **Large (minimum 5 quart) slow cooker**

2 tbsp	olive oil (approx.), divided	25 mL
2 lbs	trimmed stewing lamb, cut into 1-inch (2.5 cm) cubes	1 kg
2	onions, finely chopped	2
8	carrots, peeled and sliced	8
4	stalks celery, sliced	4
4	cloves garlic, minced	4
2 tsp	herbes de Provence	10 mL
1 tsp	salt	5 mL
½ tsp	cracked black peppercorns	2 mL
2	bay leaves	2
1 cup	lower-salt vegetable or chicken broth	250 mL
1	can (28 oz/796 mL) diced tomatoes, including juice	1
2 cups	green or brown lentils, rinsed	500 mL
8 cups	chopped stemmed Swiss chard (about 2 bunches) (see Tips, left)	2 L

1. In a skillet, heat 1 tbsp (15 mL) of the oil over medium-high heat for 30 seconds. Add lamb, in batches, and cook, stirring, adding more oil as necessary, until browned, about 4 minutes per batch. Transfer to slow cooker stoneware.

2. Reduce heat to medium. Drain all but 1 tbsp (15 mL) of the fat from pan. Add onions, carrots and celery to pan and cook, stirring, until carrots are softened, about 7 minutes. Add garlic, herbes de Provence, salt and peppercorns and cook, stirring, for 1 minute. Add bay leaves, broth and tomatoes with juice and bring to a boil, Transfer to slow cooker stoneware. Stir in lentils.

3. Cover and cook on Low for 8 hours or on High for 4 hours, until mixture is bubbly and lamb and lentils are tender. Add chard, in batches, stirring each batch into the stew until wilted. Cover and cook on High for 20 to 30 minutes, until chard is tender. Discard bay leaves.

AMERICA'S EXCHANGES	
2	Starch
3	Very Lean Meat
1	Fat

CANADA'S CHOICES	
1½	Carbohydrate
3	Meat and Alternatives

Tip

I prefer a peppery base in this dish to balance the sweetness of the apricots and raisins, so I usually use a whole teaspoon (5 mL) of cracked black peppercorns in this recipe. But I'm a pepper lover, so use your own judgment.

Moroccan-Style Lamb with Raisins and Apricots

This classic tagine-style recipe, in which lamb is braised in spices and honey, is an appetizing combination of savory and sweet. I like to serve this over couscous, preferably whole wheat, which is the traditional accompaniment. It is also delicious served with fluffy quinoa, which adds a New World twist to this Middle Eastern dish.

- **Works in slow cookers from 3½ to 6 quarts**

1 tbsp	cumin seeds	15 mL
1 tsp	coriander seeds	5 mL
2 tbsp	olive oil (approx.), divided	25 mL
2 lbs	trimmed stewing lamb, cut into 1-inch (2.5 cm) cubes	1 kg
1	onion, finely chopped	1
1 tbsp	minced gingerroot	15 mL
1 tsp	grated lemon zest	5 mL
1 tsp	salt	5 mL
½ tsp	cracked black peppercorns (approx.) (see Tip, left)	2 mL
1	piece (1 inch/2.5 cm) cinnamon stick	1
½ cup	lower-salt chicken broth	125 mL
1 tbsp	freshly squeezed lemon juice	15 mL
1 tbsp	liquid honey	15 mL
1 cup	dried apricots, chopped	250 mL
½ cup	raisins	125 mL
¼ cup	finely chopped cilantro leaves	50 mL

1. In a dry skillet over medium heat, toast cumin and coriander seeds, stirring, until fragrant and cumin seeds just begin to brown, about 3 minutes. Immediately transfer to a mortar or a spice grinder and grind. Set aside.

2. In same skillet, heat 1 tbsp (15 mL) of the oil over medium-high heat for 30 seconds. Add lamb, in batches, and cook, stirring, adding more oil as necessary, until browned, about 4 minutes per batch. Transfer to slow cooker stoneware.

NUTRIENTS PER SERVING	
Calories	246
Fat	8.7 g
Saturates	2.7 g
Polyunsaturates	0.8 g
Monounsaturates	4.1 g
Cholesterol	65 mg
Sodium	418 mg
Carbohydrate	22.5 g
Fiber	2.3 g
Protein	20.7 g

AMERICA'S EXCHANGES	
1½	Fruit
3	Lean Meat

CANADA'S CHOICES	
1	Carbohydrate
2½	Meat and Alternatives

Make Ahead

This dish can be partially prepared before it is cooked. Complete Step 1. Heat 1 tbsp (15 mL) of the oil and complete Step 3. Cover and refrigerate overnight or for up to 2 days. When you're ready to cook, either brown the lamb as outlined in Step 2 or add it to the stoneware without browning. Stir well and continue with Step 4.

3. Reduce heat to medium. Add onion to pan and cook, stirring, until softened. Add gingerroot, lemon zest, salt, peppercorns, cinnamon stick and reserved cumin and coriander and cook, stirring, for 1 minute. Add broth and bring to a boil. Transfer to slow cooker stoneware. Stir well.

4. Cover and cook on Low for 7 to 8 hours or on High for 3 to 4 hours, until lamb is tender. Add lemon juice and honey and stir well. Stir in apricots and raisins. Cover and cook on High for 20 minutes, until fruit is warmed through. Garnish with cilantro. Discard cinnamon stick.

Mindful Morsels

In addition to providing a hint of exotic flavor, the apricots in this recipe deepen its nutritional value by adding fiber, vitamin A (as beta carotene), potassium and iron. Enjoying apricots in a stew has an added benefit because their beta carotene becomes more available to the body when they are cooked. Dried apricots are available year-round and make a very nutritious snack. There's just one thing to watch for — most dried apricots are treated with sulfur dioxide, which maintains their bright orange color but can trigger allergic reactions or an asthma attack in people sensitive to sulfur. I prefer to buy sulfur-free versions at a natural foods store.

Tip

Chile nomenclature can be confusing. Long red or green chiles are usually used in Indian cooking and can be found in Asian markets. They are sometimes called cayenne or serrano chiles, not to be confused with Mexican serrano chiles, which are different.

Curried Lamb with Apples and Bananas

The spices produce a mildly flavored dish. If you like a bit of heat, add the second chile pepper or up to ¼ tsp (1 mL) cayenne (along with the chile), which nicely balances the sweetness of the fruit. Serve this over long-grain brown rice and add steamed spinach to round out the meal.

- **Works in slow cookers from 3½ to 6 quarts**

1 tbsp	cumin seeds	15 mL
1 tsp	coriander seeds	5 mL
1 tbsp	olive oil (approx.)	15 mL
2 lbs	trimmed stewing lamb, cut into 1-inch (2.5 cm) cubes	1 kg
2	onions, finely chopped	2
4	cloves garlic, minced	4
1 tbsp	minced gingerroot	15 mL
2 tsp	turmeric	10 mL
1	piece (2 inches/5 cm) cinnamon stick	1
2	black cardamom pods, crushed	2
½ tsp	cracked black peppercorns	2 mL
1 cup	lower-salt beef or chicken broth	250 mL
1 to 2	long red or green chile peppers (see Tip, left), minced, or ¼ tsp (1 mL) cayenne, dissolved in 1 tbsp (15 mL) boiling water	1 to 2
3	apples, peeled, cored and thinly sliced	3
2	bananas, thinly sliced	2
¼ cup	finely chopped cilantro or parsley leaves	50 mL

1. In a large dry skillet over medium heat, toast cumin and coriander seeds, stirring, until fragrant and cumin seeds just begin to brown, about 3 minutes. Immediately transfer to a mortar or a spice grinder and grind. Set aside.

2. In same skillet, heat oil over medium-high heat for 30 seconds. Add lamb, in batches, and cook, stirring, adding more oil if necessary, until browned, about 4 minutes per batch. Using a slotted spoon, transfer to slow cooker stoneware.

NUTRIENTS PER SERVING	
Calories	244
Fat	8.4 g
Saturates	2.5 g
Polyunsaturates	0.8 g
Monounsaturates	3.8 g
Cholesterol	73 mg
Sodium	151 mg
Carbohydrate	18.3 g
Fiber	2.2 g
Protein	24.4 g

AMERICA'S EXCHANGES	
1	Vegetable
1	Fruit
3	Lean Meat

CANADA'S CHOICES	
1	Carbohydrate
3	Meat and Alternatives

This dish can be partially prepared before it is cooked. Complete Step 1. Heat oil and complete Step 3. Cover and refrigerate for up to 2 days. When you're ready to cook, either brown the lamb (Step 2) or add it to the stoneware without browning. Stir well and continue with Step 4.

3. Reduce heat to medium. Add onions to pan and cook, stirring, until softened, about 3 minutes. Add garlic, gingerroot, turmeric, cinnamon stick, cardamom, peppercorns and reserved cumin and coriander and cook, stirring, until spices release their aroma, about 1 minute. Add broth and bring to a boil.

4. Pour sauce over lamb and stir well. Cover and cook on Low for 7 to 8 hours or on High for 3 to 4 hours, until lamb is very tender. Discard cinnamon stick and cardamom pods. Add chile peppers, apples and bananas, in batches, stirring to incorporate each batch before adding the next. Cover and cook on High for 30 minutes, until fruit is tender and hot. Garnish with cilantro.

Mindful Morsels

Most of us grew up taking it on faith that an apple a day keeps the doctor away. Now scientists are confirming the truth of this maxim and explaining the reasons why. We've long known that apples contain nutrients such as vitamin C and fiber, but it's the range of phytochemicals, such as the flavonoid quercitin (found mainly in the skin), that most interests researchers today. Quercitin is a potent antioxidant that works to strengthen the body's immune system.

Tips

To purée garlic, use a fine, sharp-toothed grater such as those made by Microplane.

Canned tomatoes vary in sizes. If your supermarket carries the 19-oz (540 mL) can of diced tomatoes, by all means substitute it in this recipe.

Not Your Granny's Pork and Beans

This dish requires a bit of advance planning because the pork is marinated overnight in a salt and garlic rub, which imbues it with deep flavor. Otherwise it is simple, straightforward and loaded with flavor. To complement the Mediterranean ingredients, I like to accompany this with a platter of marinated roasted peppers. Add warm crusty bread, such as ciabatta, and if you're feeling festive, a robust Rioja, for a perfect meal. It makes a large quantity but reheats well.

- **Works best in a large (minimum 5 quart) slow cooker**

1 tbsp	puréed garlic (see Tips, left)	15 mL
½ tsp	cracked black peppercorns	2 mL
2 lbs	trimmed boneless pork shoulder, cut into bite-size pieces	1 kg
2 tbsp	olive oil, divided	25 mL
3	onions, thinly sliced on the vertical	3
6	anchovy fillets, finely chopped	6
2 tsp	dried thyme leaves, crumbled	10 mL
1 cup	dry white wine	250 mL
1 tsp	white wine vinegar	5 mL
1	can (14 oz/398 mL) diced tomatoes, including juice (see Tips, left)	1
2	cans (each 19 oz/540 mL) white kidney or navy beans, drained and rinsed	2
1 tsp	paprika, preferably smoked, dissolved in 1 tbsp (15 mL) white wine or water	5 mL
1 cup	finely chopped parsley	250 mL
1 cup	chopped pitted kalamata olives (about 48 olives)	250 mL

1. In a bowl large enough to accommodate the pork, combine garlic and peppercorns. Add pork and toss until well coated with mixture. Cover and refrigerate overnight.

2. In a skillet, heat 1 tbsp (15 mL) of the oil over medium-high heat for 30 seconds. Pat pork dry with paper towel and cook, stirring, in batches, adding more oil as necessary, until browned, about 5 minutes per batch. Using a slotted spoon, transfer to slow cooker stoneware.

NUTRIENTS PER SERVING	
Calories	268
Fat	10.7 g
Saturates	2.6 g
Polyunsaturates	1.2 g
Monounsaturates	6.0 g
Cholesterol	55 mg
Sodium	549 mg
Carbohydrate	21.4 g
Fiber	7.6 g
Protein	22.1 g

AMERICA'S EXCHANGES	
1	Vegetable
1	Starch
3	Lean Meat

CANADA'S CHOICES	
1	Carbohydrate
3	Meat and Alternatives

Make Ahead

This dish can be partially prepared before it is cooked. Complete Step 1. Heat 1 tbsp (15 mL) of the oil and complete Step 3. Cover and refrigerate meat and onion mixtures separately for up to 2 days. When you're ready to cook, either brown the pork as outlined in Step 2 or add it to the stoneware without browning. Stir well and continue with Step 4.

3. Reduce heat to medium. Add onions and anchovies to pan and cook, stirring, until onions are softened, about 3 minutes. Add thyme and cook, stirring, for 1 minute. Add wine and vinegar and cook for 2 minutes, stirring and scraping up any brown bits on the bottom of the pan. Add tomatoes with juice and bring to a boil. Transfer to slow cooker stoneware. Add beans and stir well.

4. Cover and cook on Low for 8 to 10 hours or on High for 4 to 5 hours, until pork is very tender (it should be falling apart). Stir in paprika solution, parsley and olives. Cover and cook on High for 15 minutes, until heated through.

Mindful Morsels

Contemporary farming has changed the way we think about pork. Once dismissed by health-conscious consumers as extremely fatty, pork has become almost 50% leaner than it was just a decade ago. This makes pork, eaten in moderation, a nutritious food choice.

When preparing kale, chop off the stem, then fold the leaf in half and remove the thickest part of the vein that runs up the center of the leaf.

If you don't have kale, you can substitute an equal quantity of spinach or Swiss chard.

Spanish-Style Pork and Beans

Here's a dish that is as delicious as the best Boston baked beans but even more nutritious. Salt pork or bacon is replaced with pork shoulder, trimmed of fat, and nutrient-dense kale is added just before the dish has finished cooking. Serve this with a tossed green salad sprinkled with shredded carrots. Add crusty rolls to complete the meal.

- **Large (minimum 5 quart) slow cooker**

2 tbsp	olive oil, divided	25 mL
2 lbs	trimmed boneless pork shoulder, cut into bite-size pieces	1 kg
3	onions, finely chopped	3
4	cloves garlic, minced	4
2 tsp	dried oregano leaves, crumbled	10 mL
1 tsp	salt	5 mL
½ tsp	cracked black peppercorns	2 mL
1 cup	dry white wine or lower-salt chicken broth	250 mL
2 tsp	sherry vinegar or white wine vinegar	10 mL
1	can (28 oz/796 mL) diced tomatoes, including juice	1
2	cans (each 14 to 19 oz/398 to 540 mL) white kidney beans, drained and rinsed, or 2 cups (500 mL) dried white kidney beans, soaked, cooked and drained (see Basic Beans, page 231)	2
2 tsp	hot or mild paprika, dissolved in 2 tbsp (25 mL) dry white wine or water	10 mL
8 cups	coarsely chopped stemmed kale (about 2 bunches) (see Tips, left)	2 L

1. In a skillet, heat 1 tbsp (15 mL) of the oil over medium-high heat. Add pork, in batches, and cook, stirring, adding more oil as necessary, until browned, about 5 minutes per batch. Transfer to slow cooker stoneware.

2. Reduce heat to medium. Add onions to pan and cook, stirring, until softened, about 3 minutes. Add garlic, oregano, salt and peppercorns and cook, stirring, for 1 minute. Add wine and vinegar and cook, stirring, for 1 minute. Add tomatoes with juice and bring to a boil. Transfer to slow cooker stoneware. Add beans and stir well.

NUTRIENTS PER SERVING	
Calories	277
Fat	9.5 g
Saturates	2.6 g
Polyunsaturates	1.3 g
Monounsaturates	4.8 g
Cholesterol	57 mg
Sodium	563 mg
Carbohydrate	23.4 g
Fiber	6.9 g
Protein	25.8 g

AMERICA'S EXCHANGES	
½	Starch
1	Carbohydrate
3	Lean Meat

CANADA'S CHOICES	
1	Carbohydrate
3	Meat and Alternatives

Make Ahead

This dish can be partially prepared before it is cooked. Heat 1 tbsp (15 mL) of the oil and complete Step 2. Cover and refrigerate overnight or for up to 2 days. When you're ready to cook, either brown the pork as outlined in Step 1 or add it to the stoneware without browning. Stir well and continue with Steps 3 and 4.

3. Cover and cook on Low for 8 hours or on High for 4 hours, until pork is very tender (it should be falling apart).

4. Add paprika solution and stir well. Add kale, in batches, stirring well after each addition, until it begins to wilt. Cover and cook on High for 30 minutes, until kale is tender. Serve immediately.

Mindful Morsels

It's hard to believe this delicious stew is also so nutritious. One serving is an excellent source of vitamins A, C, B_6 and K and the minerals phosphorus, potassium, iron and zinc. It is also a good source of vitamin B_{12}, folacin and magnesium, and a source of calcium. And, if that's not beneficial enough, it contains a very high amount of dietary fiber.

Tips

A serving of this dish may seem high in calories, but it is almost a complete meal in itself and doesn't need much more to complete it.

One way of preparing collard greens for use in a stew is to cut them into a chiffonade. Remove any tough veins toward the bottom of the leaves and up the center of the lower portion of the leaf. Stack about 6 leaves in a pile. Roll them up like a cigar, then slice as thinly as you can. Repeat until all the greens are sliced.

Pass a cruet of good vinegar at the table so diners can add its bitter finish to suit their tastes.

Make Ahead

This dish can be partially prepared before it is cooked. Heat 1 tbsp (15 mL) of the oil and complete Step 2. Cover and refrigerate overnight or for up to 2 days. When you're ready to cook, brown the ribs as outlined in Step 1 and continue with Step 3.

NUTRIENTS PER SERVING	
Calories	383
Fat	16.2 g
Saturates	4.9 g
Polyunsaturates	2.0 g
Monounsaturates	7.5 g
Cholesterol	60 mg
Sodium	391 mg
Carbohydrate	38.8 g
Fiber	7.4 g
Protein	22.1 g

Ribs 'n' Greens with Wheat Berries

This dish reminds me of one of my favorite dishes from the Deep South, pot likker greens. In that down-home classic, steaming collards are cooked with a ham hock and seasoned with a splash of vinegar. Here, I've substituted pork ribs for the ham hock and added nutritious wheat berries to the pot. I like to serve this in large soup plates, accompanied by warm whole wheat rolls to soak up the tasty liquid.

- **Large (minimum 6 quart) slow cooker**

1 tbsp	olive oil	15 mL
2½ lbs	sliced country-style or side pork ribs, trimmed of fat	1.25 kg
2	onions, finely chopped	2
8	stalks celery, diced	8
2	cloves garlic, minced	2
1	piece (2 inches/5 cm) cinnamon stick	1
½ tsp	cracked black peppercorns	2 mL
2 cups	wheat berries, rinsed	500 mL
4 cups	lower-salt chicken or vegetable broth	1 L
1 tbsp	paprika, dissolved in 2 tbsp (25 mL) white wine vinegar	15 mL
8 cups	thinly sliced (chiffonade) trimmed collard greens (about 2 bunches) (see Tips, left)	2 L
	Balsamic or white wine vinegar	

1. In a skillet, heat oil over medium-high heat for 30 seconds. Add ribs, in batches, and brown on both sides, about 5 minutes per batch. Transfer to slow cooker stoneware.

2. In same skillet, reduce heat to medium and add onions and celery to pan and cook, stirring, until celery is softened, about 5 minutes. Add garlic, cinnamon stick and peppercorns and cook, stirring, for 1 minute. Add wheat berries and toss to coat. Add broth and bring to a boil. Transfer to slow cooker stoneware.

3. Cover and cook on Low for 8 hours or on High for 4 hours, until ribs are tender and falling off the bone. Add paprika solution and stir well. Add collard greens, in batches, completely submerging each batch in the liquid before adding another. Cover and cook on High for 30 minutes, until collards are·tender. Discard cinnamon stick. Pass the balsamic at the table.

AMERICA'S EXCHANGES	
2	Starch
2	Vegetable
½	High-fat Meat
½	Fat

CANADA'S CHOICES	
2	Carbohydrate
2	Meat and Alternatives
1	Fat

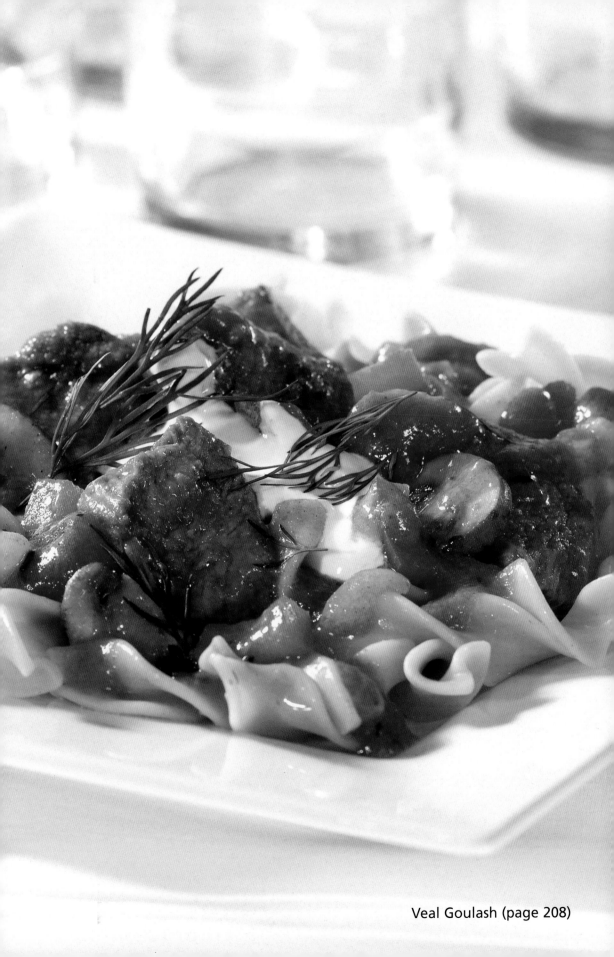

Veal Goulash (page 208)

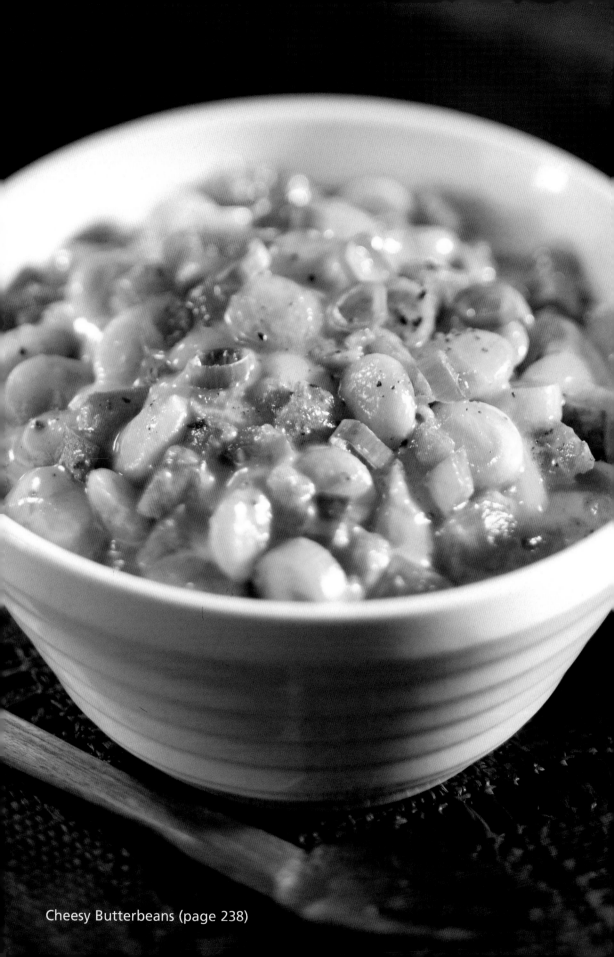

Cheesy Butterbeans (page 238)

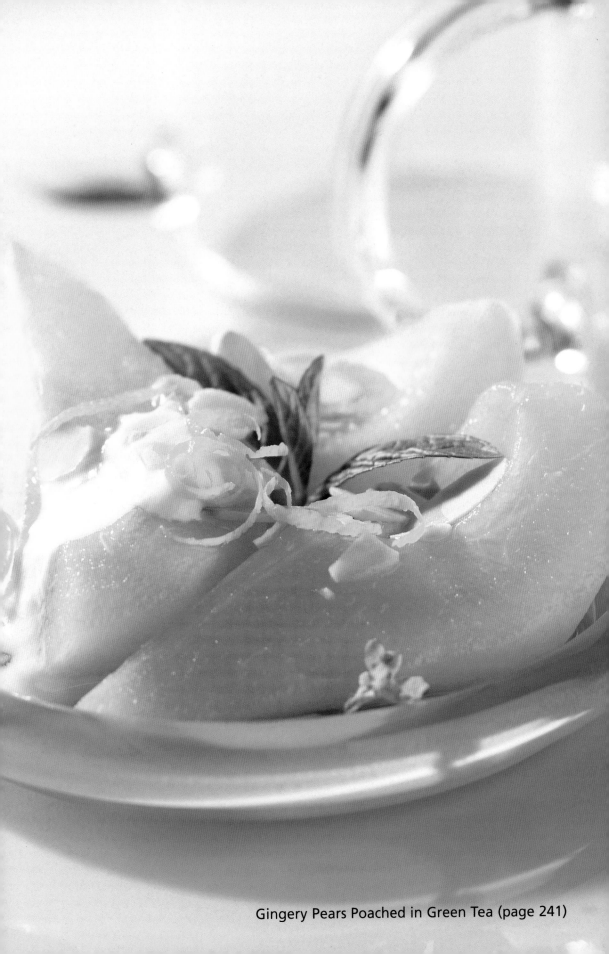

Gingery Pears Poached in Green Tea (page 241)

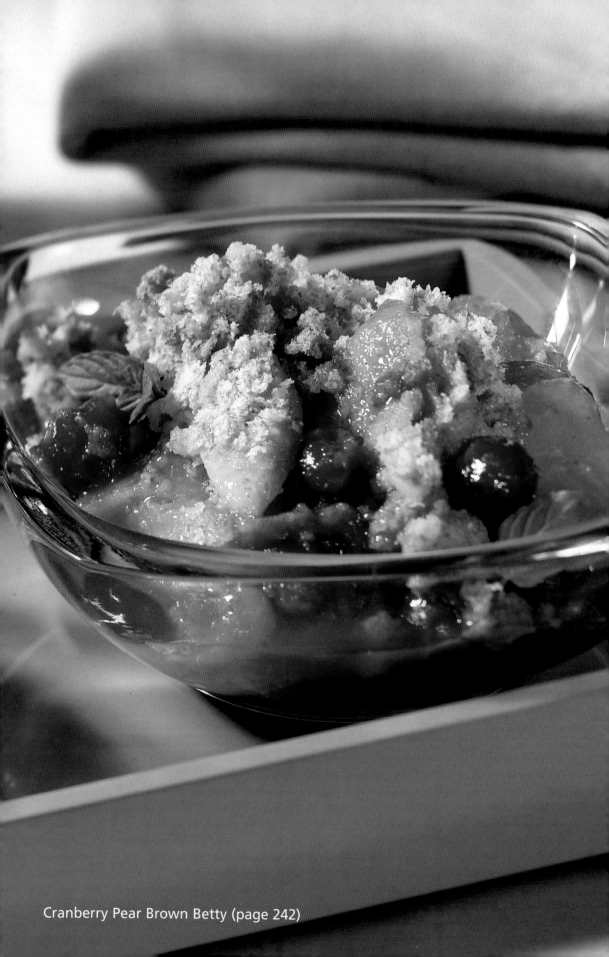

Cranberry Pear Brown Betty (page 242)

Grains and Sides

MAKES 8 SERVINGS

Tips

If using a smaller slow cooker, the cooking time will decrease to 5 to 6 hours on Low or 2½ to 3 hours on High.

To toast pine nuts: Place pine nuts in a dry skillet over medium heat. Cook, stirring constantly, until they begin to turn light gold, 3 to 4 minutes. Remove from heat and immediately transfer to a small bowl. Once they begin to brown, they can burn very quickly.

The folded tea towels absorb the moisture that accumulates during cooking, preventing it from dripping on the pilaf, which would make it soggy.

Make Ahead

This dish can be partially prepared before it is cooked. Complete Step 1. Cover and refrigerate overnight or for up to 2 days. When you're ready to cook, continue with Step 2.

Barley and Wild Rice Pilaf

Serve this tasty pilaf as a nutritious side or turn it into a light main course with the addition of a salad of sliced tomatoes or mixed greens.

- **Large (minimum 5 quart) slow cooker (see Tips, left)**

1 tbsp	olive oil	15 mL
1	onion, finely chopped	1
4	cloves garlic, minced	4
2 tsp	dried rosemary leaves, crumbled	10 mL
½ tsp	cracked black peppercorns	2 mL
1	can (28 oz/796 mL) diced tomatoes, drained	1
½ cup	wild rice	125 mL
½ cup	whole (hulled) or pot barley, rinsed	125 mL
2 cups	lower-salt vegetable or chicken broth or water	500 mL
¼ cup	toasted pine nuts (see Tips, left)	50 mL

1. In a skillet, heat oil over medium heat for 30 seconds. Add onion and cook, stirring, until softened, about 3 minutes. Add garlic, rosemary and peppercorns and cook, stirring, for 1 minute. Add tomatoes and bring to a boil. Transfer to slow cooker stoneware.

2. Add rice, barley and broth and stir well. Place two clean tea towels, each folded in half (so you will have four layers), over top of stoneware (see Tips, left). Cover and cook on Low for 8 hours or on High for 4 hours. Sprinkle with pine nuts and serve hot.

NUTRIENTS PER SERVING	
Calories	149
Fat	4.7 g
Saturates	0.8 g
Polyunsaturates	1.4 g
Monounsaturates	2.3 g
Cholesterol	0 mg
Sodium	291 mg
Carbohydrate	23.9 g
Fiber	3.2 g
Protein	4.4 g

AMERICA'S EXCHANGES	
1½	Starch
½	Fat

CANADA'S CHOICES	
1½	Carbohydrate
1	Fat

MAKES 8 SERVINGS

Rice and Bulgur Pilaf

Accompanied by a sliced tomato salad, shredded carrots in vinaigrette or a simple green salad, this tasty pilaf makes a nice weekday meal or an interesting side. It keeps warm in the slow cooker and is perfect for those evenings when everyone is coming and going at different times and can help themselves.

Tips

Don't worry if the bulgur hasn't absorbed all the water by the time you are ready to add it to the rice. Any extra will be absorbed during cooking.

To clean leeks: Fill a sink full of lukewarm water. Split the leeks in half lengthwise and submerge in water, swishing them around to remove all traces of dirt. Transfer to a colander and rinse under cold water.

Mixtures of wild and several varieties of brown rice now come in packages. Use plain brown rice instead, or you can make your own by combining ½ cup (125 mL) of each.

Make Ahead

This dish can be partially prepared before it is cooked. Complete Step 2. Cover and refrigerate overnight. The next morning, soak the bulgur (Step 1) and continue with the recipe.

- **Works best in a large (minimum 5 quart) slow cooker**

1 cup	coarse bulgur (see Tips, left)	250 mL
3 cups	boiling water	750 mL
1 tbsp	olive oil	15 mL
2	large leeks, white part only, cut in half lengthwise, cleaned and thinly sliced (see Tips, left)	2
2	stalks celery, diced	2
2	carrots, peeled and diced	2
4	cloves garlic, minced	4
1 tsp	dried thyme leaves, crumbled	5 mL
½ tsp	cracked black peppercorns	2 mL
1 cup	brown and wild rice mixture, rinsed (see Tips, left)	250 mL
¼ cup	finely chopped reconstituted sun-dried tomatoes	50 mL
2 cups	lower-salt vegetable or chicken broth	500 mL

1. In a bowl, combine bulgur and boiling water. Set aside for 20 minutes, until water is absorbed.

2. In a large skillet, heat oil over medium heat. Add leeks, celery and carrots and cook, stirring, until carrots are softened, about 7 minutes. Add garlic, thyme and peppercorns and cook, stirring, for 1 minute. Add rice and toss to coat. Add sun-dried tomatoes and stir well. Add broth, stirring, and bring to a boil.

3. Transfer to slow cooker stoneware. Stir in soaked bulgur. Place a clean tea towel, folded in half (so you will have two layers), over top of stoneware to absorb moisture. Cover and cook on High for 3 hours or on Low for 6 hours, until liquid is absorbed and rice is tender to the bite.

NUTRIENTS PER SERVING	
Calories	192
Fat	2.7 g
Saturates	0.4 g
Polyunsaturates	0.6 g
Monounsaturates	1.5 g
Cholesterol	0 mg
Sodium	188 mg
Carbohydrate	37.9 g
Fiber	5.5 g
Protein	6.0 g

AMERICA'S EXCHANGES	
2	Starch
1½	Vegetable

CANADA'S CHOICES	
2	Carbohydrate
½	Fat

MAKES 10 SERVINGS

Leek and Barley Risotto

- **Works in slow cookers from 3½ to 6 quarts**

Tip

To clean leeks: Fill sink full of lukewarm water. Split leeks in half lengthwise and submerge in water, swishing them around to remove all traces of dirt. Transfer to a colander and rinse under cold water.

Make Ahead

This dish can be partially prepared the night before it is cooked. Complete Step 1. Cover and refrigerate overnight. The next morning, continue with the recipe.

1 tbsp	olive oil	15 mL
3	leeks, white part only, cleaned and thinly sliced (see Tip, left)	3
1 tsp	salt	5 mL
½ tsp	cracked black peppercorns	2 mL
2 cups	whole (hulled), pot or pearl barley, rinsed	500 mL
1	can (28 oz/796 mL) diced tomatoes, including juice	1
3 cups	lower-salt vegetable broth or water	750 mL

1. In a skillet, heat oil over medium heat for 30 seconds. Add leeks and cook, stirring, until softened, about 5 minutes. Add salt, peppercorns and barley and cook, stirring, for 1 minute. Add tomatoes, with juice, and broth and bring to a boil. Transfer to slow cooker stoneware.

2. Cover and cook on Low for 8 hours or on High for 4 hours, until barley is tender. Serve piping hot.

NUTRIENTS PER SERVING	
Calories	160
Fat	1.9 g
Saturates	0.3 g
Polyunsaturates	0.4 g
Monounsaturates	0.9 g
Cholesterol	0 mg
Sodium	427 mg
Carbohydrate	33.9 g
Fiber	4.1 g
Protein	3.4 g

AMERICA'S EXCHANGES	
2	Starch
1	Vegetable

CANADA'S CHOICES	
2	Carbohydrate
½	Fat

MAKES 8 SERVINGS

Tip

Depending upon your preference, you can cook polenta directly in the slow cooker stoneware or in a lightly greased 6-cup (1.5 L) baking dish. If you are cooking directly in the stoneware, I recommend using a small (maximum 3½ quart) slow cooker, lightly greased. If you are using a baking dish, you will need a large (minimum 5 quart) oval slow cooker.

Make Ahead

This dish can be partially prepared before it is cooked. Complete Step 1. Transfer to a container, cover and refrigerate overnight or for up to 2 days. When you're ready to cook, continue with Step 2.

Basic Polenta

Polenta, which is cornmeal cooked in seasoned liquid, is extremely nutritious and goes well with many different foods. It is usually served as a side dish. To add variety to your diet, consider topping polenta with sauces traditionally served with pasta.

- **Works in slow cookers from 3½ to 6 quarts**

4 cups	lower-salt vegetable or chicken broth or water	1 L
½ tsp	salt	2 mL
¼ tsp	freshly ground black pepper	1 mL
1¼ cups	coarse yellow cornmeal, preferably stone-ground	300 mL

1. In a saucepan over medium heat, bring broth, salt and pepper to a boil. Add cornmeal in a thin stream, stirring constantly.

2. **Direct method:** Transfer mixture to prepared slow cooker stoneware (see Tip, left). Cover and cook on Low for 1½ hours.

3. **Baking dish method:** Transfer mixture to prepared baking dish (see Tip, left). Cover with foil and secure with a string. Place dish in slow cooker stoneware and pour in enough boiling water to come 1 inch (2.5 cm) up the sides of the dish. Cover and cook on Low for 1½ hours.

NUTRIENTS PER SERVING	
Calories	88
Fat	0.5 g
Saturates	0.1 g
Polyunsaturates	0.2 g
Monounsaturates	0.1 g
Cholesterol	0 mg
Sodium	319 mg
Carbohydrate	17.3 g
Fiber	1.6 g
Protein	3.1 g

AMERICA'S EXCHANGES	
1	Starch

CANADA'S CHOICES	
1	Carbohydrate

Creamy Polenta with Corn and Chiles

MAKES 8 SERVINGS

Tip

There are two ways to make polenta in the slow cooker. You can cook it directly in a small slow cooker, as I've done in this recipe, or in a baking dish, which is the method to use if you have a large oval slow cooker. You'll need a baking dish that fits into your stoneware, and it should be lightly greased. Transfer the hot mixture to the prepared dish, cover with foil and secure with a string. Place the dish in the stoneware and add enough boiling water to come 1 inch (2.5 cm) up the sides of the dish. Cover and cook on Low for 2 hours.

In my opinion, polenta is a quintessential comfort food. I love it as side dish, where it is particularly apt at complementing robust stews. This version contains the luscious combination of corn and chiles.

- **Works best in a small (3½ quart) slow cooker**
- **Greased slow cooker stoneware**

3 cups	skim milk	750 mL
2	cloves garlic, minced	2
1 tsp	finely chopped fresh rosemary leaves or ½ tsp (2 mL) dried rosemary leaves, crumbled	5 mL
¼ tsp	salt	1 mL
	Freshly ground black pepper	
¾ cup	coarse yellow cornmeal, preferably stone-ground	175 mL
1 cup	corn kernels	250 mL
1 cup	shredded Monterey Jack cheese	250 mL
½ cup	freshly grated Parmesan cheese	125 mL
1	can (4½ oz/127 mL) diced mild green chiles	1

1. In a large saucepan over medium heat, bring milk, garlic, rosemary, salt and black pepper to taste to a boil. Gradually add polenta, in a steady stream, whisking to remove all lumps. Continue whisking until mixture begins to thicken and bubbles like lava, about 5 minutes. Add corn, Jack and Parmesan cheeses and chiles and mix well. Transfer to slow cooker stoneware.

2. Cover and cook on Low for 2 hours, until mixture is firm and just beginning to brown around the edges.

NUTRIENTS PER SERVING	
Calories	181
Fat	6.7 g
Saturates	4.1 g
Polyunsaturates	0.3 g
Monounsaturates	1.9 g
Cholesterol	20 mg
Sodium	447 mg
Carbohydrate	19.7 g
Fiber	1.3 g
Protein	11.0 g

AMERICA'S EXCHANGES	
1	Starch
½	Milk
½	Medium-fat Meat
1	Fat

CANADA'S CHOICES	
1	Carbohydrate
1	Meat and Alternatives
1	Fat

**MAKES ABOUT
2½ CUPS (625 ML)**
(½ cup/125 mL per
serving)

Tips

This recipe may be doubled or tripled to suit the quantity of beans required for a recipe.

Once cooked, legumes should be covered and stored in the refrigerator, where they will keep for 4 to 5 days. Cooked legumes can also be frozen in an airtight container. They will keep frozen for up to 6 months.

A bouquet garni is a bundle of herbs (usually parsley, thyme and a bay leaf) tied together in cheesecloth. It is traditionally used in French cooking to add flavor to dishes.

Variation

Substitute any dried bean (for instance, red kidney beans, pinto beans, white navy beans) chickpeas, black-eyed peas or split yellow peas for the white beans. Soybeans and chickpeas take longer than other legumes to cook. They will likely take the full 12 hours on Low (about 6 hours on High).

Basic Beans

Loaded with nutrition and high in fiber, dried beans are one of our most healthful edibles. And the slow cooker excels at transforming them into potentially sublime fare. It is also extraordinarily convenient. Put presoaked beans into the slow cooker before you go to bed and in the morning they are ready for whatever recipe you intend to make.

- **Works in slow cookers from 3½ to 6 quarts**

1 cup	dried white beans	250 mL
3 cups	water	750 mL
	Bouquet garni, optional	

1. **Long soak:** In a bowl, combine beans and water. Soak for at least 6 hours or overnight. Drain and rinse thoroughly with cold water. Beans are now ready for cooking.

2. **Quick soak:** In a pot, combine beans and water. Cover and bring to a boil. Boil for 3 minutes. Turn off heat and soak for 1 hour. Drain and rinse thoroughly under cold water. Beans are now ready to cook.

3. **Cooking:** In slow cooker stoneware, combine the presoaked beans and 3 cups (750 mL) fresh cold water. If desired, season with garlic, bay leaves or a bouquet garni made from your favorite herbs tied together in a cheesecloth. Cover and cook on Low for 10 to 12 hours or overnight or on High for 5 to 6 hours, until beans are tender. Drain and rinse. If not using immediately, cover and refrigerate. The beans are now ready for use in your favorite recipe.

Dried Lentils

These instructions also work for dried lentils, with the following changes: Do not presoak them and reduce the cooking time to about 6 hours on Low.

Mindful Morsels

Beans prepared from scratch without salt contain almost no sodium. Half a cup (125 mL) of regular canned beans (even after draining and rinsing) contains about 300 mg of sodium.

NUTRIENTS PER SERVING	
Calories	129
Fat	0.3 g
Saturates	0.1 g
Polyunsaturates	0.1 g
Monounsaturates	0.0 g
Cholesterol	0 mg
Sodium	2 mg
Carbohydrate	23.6 g
Fiber	7.8 g
Protein	8.6 g

AMERICA'S EXCHANGES	
1½	Starch
1	Very Lean Meat

CANADA'S CHOICES	
1	Carbohydrate
1	Meat and Alternatives

Ratatouille

MAKES 8 SERVINGS

Tips

I use Italian San Marzano tomatoes in this recipe. They are richer and thicker and have more tomato flavor than domestic varieties. If you are using a domestic variety, add 1 tbsp (15 mL) tomato paste along with the tomatoes.

Be sure to rinse the salted eggplant thoroughly after sweating. Otherwise it will retain salt and your ratatouille will be too salty.

Ratatouille makes a great accompaniment to roast meat, or if you're a vegetarian, served over baked tofu.

- **Large (minimum 5 quart) slow cooker**
- **Preheat oven to 400°F (200°C)**
- **Rimmed baking sheet, ungreased**

2	medium eggplants (each about 12 oz/375 g), peeled and cut into 1-inch (2.5 cm) cubes	2
2 tbsp	kosher or coarse sea salt	25 mL
3 tbsp	olive oil, divided	45 mL
4	medium zucchini (about 1½ lbs/750 g total), peeled and thinly sliced	4
2	cloves garlic, minced	2
2	onions, thinly sliced	2
1 tsp	herbes de Provence	5 mL
½ tsp	salt	2 mL
½ tsp	cracked black peppercorns	2 mL
8 oz	mushrooms, sliced	250 g
1	can (28 oz/796 mL) diced tomatoes, including juices	1
2	green bell peppers, cut into ½-inch (1 cm) cubes	2
½ cup	chopped parsley or basil leaves	125 mL

1. In a colander over a sink, combine eggplant and salt. Toss to ensure eggplant is well coated and let stand for 30 minutes to 1 hour. Rinse thoroughly under cold running water. Lay a clean tea towel on a work surface. Working in batches over the sink and using your hands, squeeze liquid out of eggplant. Transfer to the tea towel. When batches are complete, roll the towel up and press down to remove remaining liquid. Transfer eggplant to prepared baking sheet and toss with 1 tbsp (15 mL) of the olive oil. Spread evenly on baking sheet. Cover with foil and bake in preheated oven until soft and fragrant, about 15 minutes. Remove from oven and transfer to slow cooker stoneware.

2. Meanwhile, heat 1 tbsp (15 mL) of the oil over medium-high heat. Add zucchini and cook, stirring, for 6 minutes. Add garlic and cook, stirring, until zucchini is soft and browned, about 1 minute. Transfer to a bowl. Cover and refrigerate.

NUTRIENTS PER SERVING	
Calories	121
Fat	5.6 g
Saturates	0.8 g
Polyunsaturates	0.7 g
Monounsaturates	3.8 g
Cholesterol	0 mg
Sodium	300 mg
Carbohydrate	17.5 g
Fiber	5.1 g
Protein	3.1 g

AMERICA'S EXCHANGES	
1	Carbohydrate
1	Fat

CANADA'S CHOICES	
1	Carbohydrate
1	Fat

Make Ahead

This dish can be partially prepared before it is cooked. Complete Steps 1 through 3. Cover and refrigerate stoneware and zucchini mixture separately overnight. The next day, continue with Step 4.

3. Reduce heat to medium. Add remaining 1 tbsp (15 mL) oil. Add onions and cook, stirring, until softened, about 3 minutes. Add herbes de Provence, salt and peppercorns and cook, stirring, about 1 minute. Add mushrooms and toss until coated. Stir in tomatoes and bring to a boil. Transfer to stoneware.

4. Cover and cook on Low for 6 to 8 hours or on High for 3 to 4 hours, until vegetables are tender. Add green peppers, reserved zucchini mixture and parsley and stir well. Cover and cook on High for 25 minutes, until peppers are tender and zucchini is heated through.

Mindful Morsels

Zucchini is a member of the summer squash family. While not a nutrient-dense vegetable, it does contain small amounts of a variety of nutrients, such as manganese, vitamin C, magnesium and potassium.

Mushroom Cholent

Make Ahead

This dish can be assembled the night before it is cooked. Using the Long Soak method, soak the beans overnight. Complete Step 2. Cover and refrigerate vegetable mixture overnight. The next morning, continue with the recipe.

Cholent made with brisket, which is prepared on Friday and left to cook overnight, is the traditional midday meal for the Jewish Sabbath. In this version, portobello mushrooms provide heartiness and a mirepoix containing parsnips, as well as the traditional vegetables, adds sweetness and flavor. The mushrooms contribute to a surprisingly rich gravy and the results are very good indeed.

- **Works best in a large (minimum 5 quart) slow cooker**

1 cup	dried white navy beans	250 mL
1 tbsp	olive oil	15 mL
2	onions, finely chopped	2
4	stalks celery, diced	4
2	carrots, peeled and diced	2
2	parsnips, peeled and diced	2
6	cloves garlic, minced	6
1 tbsp	minced gingerroot	15 mL
2 tsp	paprika	10 mL
1 tsp	salt	5 mL
1 tsp	cracked black peppercorns	5 mL
4 cups	lower-salt vegetable broth	1 L
2	potatoes, peeled and cut into ½-inch (1 cm) cubes	2
12 oz	portobello mushroom caps (about 4 large)	375 g
1 cup	whole (hulled), pot or pearl barley, rinsed	250 mL

1. Soak beans according to either method in Basic Beans (see page 231). Drain and rinse and set aside.

2. In a skillet, heat oil over medium heat for 30 seconds. Add onions, celery, carrots and parsnips and cook, stirring, until softened, about 7 minutes. Add garlic, gingerroot, paprika, salt and peppercorns and cook, stirring for 1 minute. Stir in broth and remove from heat.

NUTRIENTS PER SERVING	
Calories	184
Fat	2.0 g
Saturates	0.3 g
Polyunsaturates	0.4 g
Monounsaturates	0.9 g
Cholesterol	0 mg
Sodium	371 mg
Carbohydrate	36.7 g
Fiber	6.3 g
Protein	6.5 g

AMERICA'S EXCHANGES	
1	Starch
½	Vegetable
1	Other Carbohydrate
½	Very Lean Meat

CANADA'S CHOICES	
2	Carbohydrate
½	Meat and Alternatives

3. Pour half the contents of pan into slow cooker stoneware. Set remainder aside. Spread potatoes evenly over mixture. Arrange mushrooms evenly over potatoes, cutting one to fit, if necessary. Spread barley and reserved beans evenly over mushrooms. Add remaining onion mixture to stoneware.

4. Cover and cook on Low for 10 to 12 hours or on High for 5 to 6 hours, until beans are tender.

Mindful Morsels

To maximize your intake of nutrients when making this recipe, be sure to use whole (hulled) barley rather than pearl barley, from which the germ and most of the bran has been removed. If you can find it, hull-less barley, an heirloom whole grain variety, will also work well in this recipe. Look for whole grain barley and other whole grains in natural food stores or specialty purveyors such as Whole Foods. Although supermarkets are increasing their supply of whole grains, most of the grains they stock are refined. Refined grains may be subsequently enriched with the addition of nutrients such as niacin, riboflavin, thiamin and iron, but they lack the full range of nutrients found in whole grains, and they provide less fiber.

MAKES 8 SERVINGS

Tips

To toast cumin seeds: In a dry skillet over medium heat, toast cumin seeds, stirring, until fragrant and seeds just begin to brown, about 3 minutes. Immediately transfer to a spice grinder or mortar, or use the bottom of a measuring cup or wine bottle to coarsely grind.

If you prefer not to use sugar, you may substitute your favorite low-calorie sweetener.

Make Ahead

Peel and cut parsnips and carrots. Cover and refrigerate overnight.

Parsnip and Carrot Purée with Cumin

The cumin adds a slightly exotic note to this traditional dish, which makes a great accompaniment to many foods.

• **Works in slow cookers from 3½ to 6 quarts**

4 cups	cubed peeled parsnips (½-inch/1 cm cubes)	1 L
2 cups	thinly sliced peeled carrots	500 mL
1 tsp	cumin seeds, toasted and coarsely ground (see Tips, left)	5 mL
1 tbsp	butter or butter substitute	15 mL
1 tsp	granulated sugar	5 mL
½ tsp	salt	2 mL
¼ tsp	freshly ground black pepper	1 mL
¼ cup	water or lower-salt vegetable broth	50 mL

1. In slow cooker stoneware, combine parsnips, carrots, toasted cumin, butter or butter substitute, sugar, salt, pepper and water. Cover and cook on Low for 8 to 10 hours or on High for 4 to 5 hours, until vegetables are tender.

2. Using a potato masher or a food processor or blender, mash or purée mixture until smooth. Serve immediately.

NUTRIENTS PER SERVING	
Calories	85
Fat	1.8 g
Saturates	1.0 g
Polyunsaturates	0.1 g
Monounsaturates	0.5 g
Cholesterol	4 mg
Sodium	188 mg
Carbohydrate	17.3 g
Fiber	3.2 g
Protein	1.3 g

AMERICA'S EXCHANGES	
2	Vegetable
½	Other Carbohydrate

CANADA'S CHOICES	
1	Carbohydrate

MAKES 8 SERVINGS

Make Ahead

This dish can be partially prepared before it is cooked. Complete Step 1. Cover and refrigerate overnight. The next morning, continue with the recipe.

Saffron-Scented Fennel Gratin

This flavorful gratin is a great accompaniment to roast chicken or beef.

• **Works in slow cookers from 3½ to 6 quarts**

2 tbsp	olive oil	25 mL
3	bulbs fennel, trimmed, cored and thinly sliced on the vertical	3
2 cups	lower-salt vegetable broth	500 mL
	Freshly ground black pepper, optional	
½ tsp	saffron threads	2 mL
½ cup	coarsely grated Parmesan cheese	125 mL

1. In a skillet, heat oil over medium-high heat for 30 seconds. Add fennel, in batches, adding more oil as necessary, and cook, stirring, just until the fennel begins to brown, about 5 minutes per batch. Transfer to slow cooker stoneware and add broth. Season to taste with pepper, if using.

2. Place a clean tea towel, folded in half (so you will have two layers), over top of stoneware to absorb moisture. Cover and cook on Low for 6 hours or on High for 3 hours, until fennel is tender.

3. Preheat broiler. Using a slotted spoon, transfer fennel to a heatproof serving dish and cover. Pour liquid from slow cooker into a saucepan and add saffron. Bring to a boil over medium heat and cook until reduced by half, about 6 minutes. Pour over fennel. Sprinkle with Parmesan and place under broiler until cheese is melted and brown.

NUTRIENTS PER SERVING	
Calories	93
Fat	5.6 g
Saturates	1.7 g
Polyunsaturates	0.3 g
Monounsaturates	3.0 g
Cholesterol	5 mg
Sodium	277 mg
Carbohydrate	7.9 g
Fiber	3.0 g
Protein	3.9 g

AMERICA'S EXCHANGES	
1½	Vegetable
1	Fat

CANADA'S CHOICES	
½	Meat and Alternatives
1	Fat
1	Extra

MAKES 8 SERVINGS

Cheesy Butterbeans

Make Ahead

This dish can be partially prepared before it is cooked. Complete Step 1. Cover and refrigerate overnight. The next morning, continue with the recipe.

Serve these tasty beans with grilled or roasted meat or add a salad and enjoy them as a light main course.

• **Works in slow cookers from 3½ to 6 quarts**

4 cups	frozen lima beans, thawed and drained	1 L
1	can (28 oz/796 mL) diced tomatoes, drained, ½ cup (125 mL) of the juice set aside	1
½ cup	chopped green onions	125 mL
1 tsp	salt	5 mL
	Freshly ground black pepper	
1	green bell pepper, chopped	1
1 cup	shredded light old Cheddar cheese	250 mL

1. In slow cooker stoneware, combine beans, tomatoes, ½ cup (125 mL) tomato juice, green onions, salt and black pepper to taste.

2. Cover and cook on Low for 6 hours or on High for 3 hours, until hot and bubbly. Stir in green pepper and cheese. Cover and cook on High for 20 minutes, until pepper is tender and cheese is melted.

NUTRIENTS PER SERVING	
Calories	158
Fat	3.5 g
Saturates	2.1 g
Polyunsaturates	0.2 g
Monounsaturates	0.1 g
Cholesterol	10 mg
Sodium	572 mg
Carbohydrate	22.2 g
Fiber	4.6 g
Protein	10.2 g

AMERICA'S EXCHANGES	
1	Starch
1	Vegetable
1	Lean Meat

CANADA'S CHOICES	
1	Carbohydrate
1	Meat and Alternatives

Desserts

MAKES 8 SERVINGS

MAKES 8 SERVINGS

Tip

Buy nuts from a store with high turnover. They are high in fat and tend to become rancid very quickly. This is especially true of walnuts. Taste before you buy. If they are not sweet, substitute an equal quantity of pecans.

The Ultimate Baked Apples

These luscious apples, simple to make yet delicious, are the definitive autumn dessert. I like to serve these with a dollop of whipped cream, but they are equally delicious (and healthier) accompanied by yogurt or on their own.

- **Large (minimum 5 quart) oval slow cooker**

½ cup	chopped toasted walnuts (see Tip, left)	125 mL
½ cup	dried cranberries	125 mL
2 tbsp	packed brown sugar	25 mL
1 tsp	grated orange zest	5 mL
8	apples, cored	8
1 cup	cranberry juice (no sugar added)	250 mL
	Low-fat vanilla-flavored yogurt or whipped cream, optional	

1. In a bowl, combine walnuts, cranberries, brown sugar and orange zest. To stuff the apples, hold your hand over the bottom of the apple and, using your fingers, tightly pack core space with filling. One at a time, place filled apples in slow cooker stoneware. Drizzle cranberry juice evenly over tops.

2. Cover and cook on Low for 8 hours or on High for 4 hours, until apples are tender. Transfer to a serving dish and spoon cooking juices over them. Serve hot with a dollop of yogurt, if using.

NUTRIENTS PER SERVING	
Calories	180
Fat	5.5 g
Saturates	0.6 g
Polyunsaturates	3.7 g
Monounsaturates	0.7 g
Cholesterol	0 mg
Sodium	2 mg
Carbohydrate	35.6 g
Fiber	4.0 g
Protein	1.4 g

AMERICA'S EXCHANGES	
2½	Fruit
1	Fat

CANADA'S CHOICES	
2	Carbohydrate
1	Fat

MAKES 8 SERVINGS

Tips

I prefer a strong ginger taste in these pears, but some might feel it overpowers the taste of the pears. Vary the amount of ginger to suit your preference.

When poaching, use firmer pears, such as Bosc, for best results.

Make Ahead

This dessert should be made early in the day or the night before so it can be well chilled before serving.

Gingery Pears Poached in Green Tea

I love the combination of ginger and pears in this light but delicious dessert. Sprinkle with toasted almonds and top with a dollop of vanilla yogurt for a perfect finish to a substantial meal.

- **Works best in a small (3½ quart) slow cooker**

4 cups	boiling water	1 L
2 tbsp	green tea leaves	25 mL
1 to 2 tbsp	grated gingerroot (see Tips, left)	15 to 25 mL
½ cup	liquid honey	125 mL
1 tsp	almond extract	5 mL
1 tsp	grated lemon zest	5 mL
8	firm pears, such as Bosc, peeled, cored and cut into quarters lengthwise	8
	Toasted sliced almonds, optional	
	Low-fat vanilla-flavored yogurt, optional	

1. In a pot, combine boiling water and green tea leaves. Cover and let steep for 5 minutes. Strain through a fine sieve into slow cooker stoneware.

2. Add gingerroot, honey, almond extract and lemon zest and stir well. Add pears. Cover and cook on Low for 6 hours or on High for 3 hours, until pears are tender. Transfer to a serving bowl, cover and chill thoroughly. Serve garnished with toasted almonds and a dollop of yogurt, if using.

NUTRIENTS PER SERVING	
Calories	131
Fat	0.5 g
Saturates	0.0 g
Polyunsaturates	0.1 g
Monounsaturates	0.1 g
Cholesterol	0 mg
Sodium	1 mg
Carbohydrate	34.5 g
Fiber	2.4 g
Protein	0.5 g

AMERICA'S EXCHANGES	
1	Fruit
1	Other Carbohydrate

CANADA'S CHOICES	
2	Carbohydrate

Cranberry Pear Brown Betty

MAKES 8 SERVINGS

Tips

To make dried bread crumbs for this recipe, toast 4 slices of whole wheat bread. Tear into pieces and process in a food processor fitted with a metal blade until finely ground.

Use a light-tasting whole wheat loaf for this recipe. Those with heavy molasses content will overpower the fruit.

I love the combination of textures and flavors in this old-fashioned favorite. When cranberries are in season, I always freeze a bag or two so I can make this wholesome dessert year-round. It's a great way to use up day-old bread.

- **Works best in a small (3½ quart) slow cooker**
- **Greased slow cooker stoneware**

2 cups	dry coarse whole wheat bread crumbs (see Tips, left)	500 mL
2 tbsp	butter, melted, or extra virgin olive oil	25 mL
6	pears, peeled, cored and sliced	6
1 tbsp	freshly squeezed lemon juice	15 mL
1 cup	fresh or frozen cranberries	250 mL
¼ cup	packed brown sugar	50 mL
½ cup	cranberry cocktail (no sugar added)	125 mL

1. In a bowl, combine bread crumbs and butter. Set aside.

2. In a separate bowl, combine pears, lemon juice, cranberries and brown sugar.

3. In prepared slow cooker stoneware, spread one-third of the bread crumb mixture. Layer half of the pear mixture over top. Repeat. Finish with a layer of crumbs and pour cranberry cocktail over top. Cover and cook on High for 4 hours, until fruit is tender and mixture is hot and bubbly.

NUTRIENTS PER SERVING	
Calories	150
Fat	3.8 g
Saturates	1.9 g
Polyunsaturates	0.3 g
Monounsaturates	1.1 g
Cholesterol	8 mg
Sodium	85 mg
Carbohydrate	30.3 g
Fiber	4.4 g
Protein	1.5 g

AMERICA'S EXCHANGES	
1	Starch
1	Fruit
½	Fat

CANADA'S CHOICES	
2	Carbohydrate
½	Fat

MAKES 8 SERVINGS

Tips

To make dried bread crumbs for this recipe, toast 4 slices of whole wheat bread. Tear into pieces and process in a food processor fitted with a metal blade until finely ground.

Use a light-flavored whole wheat loaf for this recipe. Those with heavy molasses content will overpower the fruit.

Peach Raspberry Betty

The combination of peaches and raspberries is a personal favorite. Although I enjoy making this dessert in summer when fresh fruit is in season, it is also delicious made with canned and/or frozen fruit, making it a year-round treat.

- **Works in slow cookers from 3½ to 6 quarts**
- **Lightly greased slow cooker stoneware**

2 cups	dry whole wheat bread crumbs (see Tips, left)	500 mL
¼ cup	chopped toasted almonds	50 mL
2 tbsp	extra virgin olive or coconut oil or almond butter	25 mL
5 cups	sliced peaches (about 4 or 5)	1.25 L
2 cups	raspberries	500 mL
½ cup	packed brown sugar	125 mL
1 tbsp	all-purpose flour	15 mL
½ tsp	almond extract	2 mL
¼ cup	cranberry-raspberry or cranberry cocktail (no sugar added)	50 mL

1. In a bowl, combine bread crumbs, almonds and oil. Set aside.

2. In a separate bowl, combine peaches, raspberries, brown sugar, flour and almond extract.

3. In prepared slow cooker stoneware, layer one-third of the bread crumb mixture, then one-half of the peach mixture. Repeat layers of bread crumbs and fruit, then finish with a layer of bread crumbs on top. Drizzle cranberry cocktail over the top. Cover and cook on High for 2½ to 3 hours, until hot and bubbly.

NUTRIENTS PER SERVING	
Calories	200
Fat	6.1 g
Saturates	0.8 g
Polyunsaturates	1.1 g
Monounsaturates	4.0 g
Cholesterol	0 mg
Sodium	65 mg
Carbohydrate	36.5 g
Fiber	4.7 g
Protein	3.1 g

AMERICA'S EXCHANGES	
1	Starch
1	Fruit
½	Other Carbohydrate
1	Fat

CANADA'S CHOICES	
2	Carbohydrate
1	Fat

MAKES 10 SERVINGS

Tips

Cook ²⁄₃ cup (150 mL) raw rice to get the 2 cups (500 mL) of cooked rice required for this recipe.

If you prefer, use 1¹⁄₂ tsp (7 mL) pumpkin pie spice instead of the cinnamon, nutmeg and cloves.

Pumpkin Rice Pudding

The combination of flavors and the chewy but crunchy texture of this luscious pudding make it hard to resist.

- **Works best in a small (3¹⁄₂ quart) slow cooker**
- **Greased slow cooker stoneware**

2 cups	cooked brown rice (see Tips, left)	500 mL
1¹⁄₂ cups	pumpkin purée (not pie filling)	375 mL
1 cup	dried cranberries or dried cherries	250 mL
1 cup	evaporated skim milk	250 mL
¹⁄₂ cup	packed dark brown sugar	125 mL
2	eggs	2
1 tsp	ground cinnamon (see Tips, left)	5 mL
¹⁄₂ tsp	grated nutmeg	2 mL
¹⁄₄ tsp	ground cloves	1 mL
	Low-fat vanilla-flavored yogurt, whipped cream or whipped topping, optional	

1. In prepared slow cooker stoneware, combine rice, pumpkin purée and cranberries.

2. In a bowl, whisk together milk, brown sugar, eggs, cinnamon, nutmeg and cloves until smooth and blended. Stir into pumpkin mixture. Cover and cook on High for 3 hours, until pudding is set. Serve warm. Garnish with 1 tbsp (15 mL) yogurt, if using.

NUTRIENTS PER SERVING	
Calories	179
Fat	1.6 g
Saturates	0.6 g
Polyunsaturates	0.3 g
Monounsaturates	0.6 g
Cholesterol	38 mg
Sodium	54 mg
Carbohydrate	38.0 g
Fiber	2.7 g
Protein	5.0 g

AMERICA'S EXCHANGES	
¹⁄₂	Starch
1	Fruit
1	Other Carbohydrate

CANADA'S CHOICES	
2	Carbohydrate
1	Extra

Basmati Rice Pudding

MAKES 10 SERVINGS

Tip

Although brown rice is more nutritious than white rice, it is also more perishable because the germ layer contains healthful oils. Like most whole grains, it turns rancid if not properly stored. That means it's important to buy from a source with high turnover. If possible, smell before buying. It should have a fresh, nutty flavor with no hint of bitterness. Store brown rice in a cool, dry place and use within a month of purchase. Or cover tightly and refrigerate.

The cardamom in this pudding provides an irresistible Indian flavor. I like to serve it at room temperature, but it also works warm or cold. If you're feeling indulgent, add a little cream.

- **Works best in a small (3½ quart) slow cooker**
- **Lightly greased slow cooker stoneware**

4 cups	whole milk or enriched rice milk	1 L
⅓ cup	Demerara sugar	75 mL
2 tsp	ground cardamom	10 mL
¾ cup	brown basmati rice, rinsed	175 mL

1. In a large saucepan over medium heat, bring milk to a boil, stirring often. Add sugar and cardamom. Remove from heat and stir in rice. Transfer to prepared slow cooker stoneware.

2. Place a tea towel folded in half (so you will have two layers) over top of stoneware to absorb moisture. Cover and cook on High for 3 hours, until rice is tender and pudding is creamy. Transfer to a serving bowl and cool to room temperature.

NUTRIENTS PER SERVING	
Calories	138
Fat	3.7 g
Saturates	2.1 g
Polyunsaturates	0.2 g
Monounsaturates	1.0 g
Cholesterol	14 mg
Sodium	50 mg
Carbohydrate	22.0 g
Fiber	0.8 g
Protein	4.5 g

AMERICA'S EXCHANGES	
½	Starch
½	Other Carbohydrate
½	Whole Milk

CANADA'S CHOICES	
1½	Carbohydrate
½	Fat

MAKES 10 SERVINGS

Tip

Oats, in the form of oatmeal, are the most popular whole grain in North America, largely because, unlike other whole grains, they do not need to be refined to enjoy a relatively long shelf life. Oats contain a natural chemical that acts as a preservative, which means that normal processing consists of hulling and roasting, which leaves the bran and germ intact.

Apple Oatmeal Pudding

This tasty pudding, which combines luscious apples with hearty oatmeal, is an adaptation of a traditional Irish recipe.

- **Works best in a small (3½ quart) slow cooker**
- **Greased slow cooker stoneware**

2 tbsp	melted butter or extra virgin olive oil	25 mL
1 cup	rolled oats (not quick-cooking)	250 mL
⅓ cup	Demerara sugar	75 mL
½ cup	all-purpose flour	125 mL
1 tsp	baking soda	5 mL
2	eggs, beaten	2
1 cup	rice milk	250 mL
6	apples, peeled, cored and thinly sliced	6
1 tbsp	freshly squeezed lemon juice	15 mL
1 tsp	ground cinnamon	5 mL
1 tbsp	packed brown sugar	15 mL

1. In a bowl, mix together butter, oats and sugar. Stir in flour and baking soda. Gradually add eggs and rice milk, mixing until blended. Spoon into prepared slow cooker stoneware.

2. In a separate bowl, combine apples, lemon juice, cinnamon and brown sugar. Spread evenly over oatmeal mixture. Cover and cook on High for 3½ to 4 hours, until apples are tender.

NUTRIENTS PER SERVING	
Calories	177
Fat	4.4 g
Saturates	1.9 g
Polyunsaturates	0.6 g
Monounsaturates	1.3 g
Cholesterol	43 mg
Sodium	102 mg
Carbohydrate	32.4 g
Fiber	2.7 g
Protein	3.2 g

AMERICA'S EXCHANGES	
2	Starch
1	Fruit
½	Fat

CANADA'S CHOICES	
2	Carbohydrate
1	Fat

MAKES 8 SERVINGS

Cornmeal Pudding

This old-fashioned dessert is delicious served with fresh berries.

Tip

The nutrient analysis on this recipe was done using 2% milk. If you are concerned about your fat intake, use skim milk instead.

- **Works best in a small (3½ quart) slow cooker**
- **Greased slow cooker stoneware**

4 cups	2% milk (see Tip, left)	1 L
½ cup	yellow cornmeal, preferably stone-ground	125 mL
2	eggs, beaten	2
1 tbsp	extra virgin olive oil	15 mL
½ cup	fancy molasses	125 mL
½ tsp	ground ginger	2 mL
½ tsp	ground cinnamon	2 mL
½ tsp	freshly grated nutmeg	2 mL
½ tsp	salt	2 mL
	Fresh berries, optional	
	Vanilla ice cream, optional	
	Whipped cream, optional	

1. In a saucepan, heat milk over medium-high heat, stirring often to prevent scorching, until boiling. Gradually whisk in cornmeal in a steady stream. Cook, stirring, until mixture begins to thicken and bubbles like lava, about 5 minutes. Remove from heat.

2. In a small bowl, combine beaten eggs with about ½ cup (125 mL) of the hot cornmeal, beating until combined. Gradually return to pot, mixing well. Stir in olive oil, molasses, ginger, cinnamon, nutmeg and salt. Transfer to prepared slow cooker stoneware.

3. Cover and cook on High for 3 hours, until set. Spoon into individual serving bowls and top with fresh berries, vanilla ice cream or a dollop of whipped cream, if using.

NUTRIENTS PER SERVING	
Calories	181
Fat	5.5 g
Saturates	2.1 g
Polyunsaturates	0.5 g
Monounsaturates	2.4 g
Cholesterol	56 mg
Sodium	227 mg
Carbohydrate	27.0 g
Fiber	0.5 g
Protein	6.4 g

AMERICA'S EXCHANGES	
1	Starch
1	Other Carbohydrate
1	Fat

CANADA'S CHOICES	
2	Carbohydrate
1	Fat

Library and Archives Canada Cataloguing in Publication

Finlayson, Judith
    The best diabetes slow cooker recipes / Judith Finlayson ;
Barbara Selley, nutrition editor.

Includes index.
ISBN 978-0-7788-0169-6

1. Diabetes—Diet therapy—Recipes. 2. Electric cookery, Slow.
I. Selley, Barbara. II. Title.

RC662.F548 2007   641.5'6314   C2007-903176-5

Finlayson, Judith
    Canadian diabetes slow cooker recipes / Judith Finlayson,
Barbara Selley.

Includes index.
ISBN 978-0-7788-0172-6

1. Diabetes—Diet therapy—Recipes. 2. Electric cookery, Slow.
I. Selley, Barbara. II. Title.

RC662.F55 2007   641.5'6314   C2007-902981-7

Index

C

T